W0007171

THE
NURSE'S
ANATOMY,
PHYSIOLOGY AND
PATHOPHYSIOLOGY
GLOSSARY

Sara Miller McCune founded SAGE Publishing in 1965 to support the dissemination of usable knowledge and educate a global community. SAGE publishes more than 1000 journals and over 800 new books each year, spanning a wide range of subject areas. Our growing selection of library products includes archives, data, case studies and video. SAGE remains majority owned by our founder and after her lifetime will become owned by a charitable trust that secures the company's continued independence.

Los Angeles | London | New Delhi | Singapore | Washington DC | Melbourne

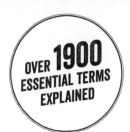

OVER **1900** ESSENTIAL TERMS EXPLAINED

NEAL COOK
ANDREA SHEPHERD
JENNIFER BOORE
STEPHANIE DUNLEAVY

THE NURSE'S ANATOMY, PHYSIOLOGY AND PATHOPHYSIOLOGY GLOSSARY

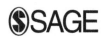

Los Angeles I London I New Delhi
Singapore I Washington DC I Melbourne

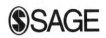

Los Angeles | London | New Delhi
Singapore | Washington DC | Melbourne

SAGE Publications Ltd
1 Oliver's Yard
55 City Road
London EC1Y 1SP

SAGE Publications Inc.
2455 Teller Road
Thousand Oaks, California 91320

SAGE Publications India Pvt Ltd
B 1/I 1 Mohan Cooperative Industrial Area
Mathura Road
New Delhi 110 044

SAGE Publications Asia-Pacific Pte Ltd
3 Church Street
#10-04 Samsung Hub
Singapore 049483

Editor: Alex Clabburn
Assistant editor: Jade Grogan
Production editor: Tanya Szwarnowska
Marketing manager: George Kimble
Cover design: Shaun Mercier
Typeset by: C&M Digitals (P) Ltd, Chennai, India
Printed in the UK

Library of Congress Control Number:
2019933544

British Library Cataloguing in Publication data

A catalogue record for this book is available from
the British Library

ISBN 978-1-5297-0109-8
ISBN 978-1-5264-9620-1 (pbk)

At SAGE we take sustainability seriously. Most of our products are printed in the UK using responsibly
sourced papers and boards. When we print overseas we ensure sustainable papers are used as
measured by the PREPS grading system. We undertake an annual audit to monitor our sustainability.

CONTENTS

ABOUT THE AUTHORS

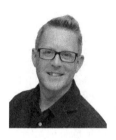

Dr Neal Cook is a Reader and the Associate Head of School at the School of Nursing, Ulster University and a Fellow of the Higher Education Academy. He is the Athena SWAN Champion for the School. He is also President of the European Association of Neuroscience Nurses and an Executive Board Member of the British Association of Neuroscience Nurses. Neal has taught anatomy, physiology and pathophysiology to undergraduate and postgraduate nursing students across a number of courses since he commenced working in higher education. Neal is also an Advanced Life Support Instructor, teaching life support courses in Health and Social Care Trusts and in the University. He has worked in the fields of neurosciences and critical care since registering as a nurse, becoming a specialist practitioner and subsequently moving into education and research. Neal has

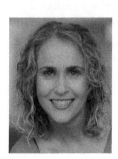

published clinical, research and education papers in the fields of education and neurosciences and is still very active in these endeavours. He remains clinically active in neurosciences and is a Registered Nurse with the Nursing and Midwifery Council (UK).

Andrea Shepherd is a Lecturer in Nursing at the School of Nursing, Ulster University and a Fellow of the

Higher Education Academy. She has taught anatomy, physiology and pathophysiology to undergraduate and postgraduate nursing students across a number of courses since she commenced working in higher education. Andrea is also an Advanced Life Support Instructor, teaching life support courses in Health and Social Care Trusts and in the University. She has worked in the fields of critical care and orthopaedics since registering as a nurse, becoming a specialist practitioner and subsequently moving into education. She currently takes a lead role in adult pre-registration nursing, is clinically active in critical care and remains a Registered Nurse with the Nursing and Midwifery Council (UK).

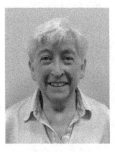

Professor Jennifer Boore is Emeritus Professor of Nursing at the School of Nursing, Ulster University. Jenny started her career as a registered nurse, and then qualified as a midwife. She practised as a nurse and midwife in the UK and Australia for some years before returning and beginning her first degree in human biology. After working as a clinical teacher with the degree students she obtained a Research Fellowship at the University of Manchester and completed her PhD on pre-operative preparation of patients. From 1977 to 1984 Jenny worked as a Lecturer in Nursing at the Universities of Edinburgh and Hull and was then appointed as Professor of Nursing at the University of Ulster in 1984 (the first Professor of Nursing in Ireland). Jenny has an extensive background in education, research and professional regulation. She has taught anatomy, physiology and pathophysiology to undergraduate and post-graduate nursing students across a number of courses throughout her career. Her contributions to nursing have been recognised in achieving the honours of Fellow of the Royal College of Nursing in 1993 and Officer of the Order of the British Empire in 1996. Jenny continues to be active in nursing education and writing.

Stephanie Dunleavy is a Lecturer in Nursing and academic lead for pre-registration Nursing programmes at the School of Nursing, Ulster University and a Fellow of the Higher Education

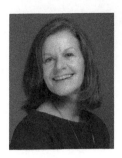

Academy. She has taught anatomy, physiology and pathophysiology to undergraduate and postgraduate nursing students across a number of courses since she commenced working in higher education. Stephanie is also an Immediate Life Support Instructor, teaching life support courses in the School. She has worked in the fields of critical care and neurosciences and has completed a BSc (Hons) in Life Sciences and a Masters of Business Administration since registering as a nurse, subsequently moving into education. She currently takes a lead role in adult pre-registration nursing and curriculum design, and remains a Registered Nurse with the Nursing and Midwifery Council (UK).

Ulster University

The School of Nursing at Ulster provides pre-registration and post-registration nursing education across two campuses in Northern Ireland and internationally. The Person-Centred Nursing Framework (McCormack and McCance, 2010) and Person-Centred Practice Framework (McCormack and McCance, 2017) inform the curricular framework for pre-registration nursing courses at the School and influence a wide variety of programmes and research activity within the School and the Institute of Nursing and Health Research. Both the School and the Institute of Nursing and Health Research are recognised as excellent and leaders in their field nationally and internationally.

McCormack, B. and McCance, T. (eds) (2010) *Person-centred Nursing: Theory and Practice (1st Edition)*. Chichester: Wiley-Blackwell.

McCormack, B. and McCance, T. (eds) (2017) *Person-centred Practice in Nursing and Health Care: Theory and Practice (2nd Edition)*. Chichester: Wiley-Blackwell.

PUBLISHER'S ACKNOWLEDGEMENTS

The publishers are grateful to the academic lecturers from the below institutions, and the nursing students from Birmingham City University and the University of Derby who reviewed the idea for a glossary. All have provided insightful and critical feedback which has shaped the book for the better.

Lecturers

Terry Ferns, University of Greenwich

Alan Monaghan, Brighton University

Andy Powell, Birmingham City University

Basem Al-Omari, Northumbria University

Students

Karen Bernard

Deborah Brennan

Danielle Carlisle

Katie Dixon

Jennifer Giampaoli

Melissa Heslop

Leona Hill

Sarah-Louise Priest

Toni Wade

INTRODUCTION

Knowledge of anatomy, physiology and pathophysiology is fundamental to being an effective and safe nurse. Nurses need to have a thorough understanding of the normal functioning of a healthy individual as well as to understand pathophysiological processes. Indeed, the Standards of Proficiency for Registered Nurses (NMC 2018: 14) state that all registered nurses should be able to 'demonstrate and apply knowledge of body systems and homeostasis, human anatomy and physiology, biology, genomics, pharmacology and social and behavioural sciences when undertaking full and accurate person-centred nursing assessments and developing appropriate care plans.' Unsurprisingly, learning the bioscience of health and illness, alongside its application in a person-centred approach, will form a major pillar of your nursing education.

Learning these subjects is challenging. It represents a new language to many students, a language that is often difficult to pronounce and with many new words/terms that are not easy to remember off hand. Tools that can support learning, refresh memory and dissect terms into their components are vitally important to students and practitioners alike. In the same way that a phrase book or dictionary can help someone learn a foreign language, a detailed glossary of biological terms can unlock the language of healthcare practice. It is fair to say that the majority of nursing students begin their studies with limited prior knowledge of the biosciences and are initially met with an array of unfamiliar terminology causing a barrier to learning. Having a firm grasp of bioscience language is also central to effective interprofessional communication. Indeed, while the terms are often challenging for people in practice to understand, nurses must understand the language sufficiently well to be able to explain them to people in their care and colleagues who may have far less knowledge of the subject. In many cases you will need to act as translator, providing accurate biological

Nursing and Midwifery Council (2018) *Standards of proficiency for registered nurses.* London: NMC

explanations about different conditions or treatments using simple language that anyone can follow.

This glossary book has been developed to help you fulfil this aspect of the nursing role. It aims to:

- provide a thorough and detailed source of information covering the major terminology for anatomy, physiology and pathophysiology
- assist with memorisation and knowledge retention
- offer a portable and practical resource to not only aid access to definitions of terms but assist in pronunciation
- provide a learning resource appropriate for student nurses that is quick, simple and effective.

This glossary is structured in three parts to achieve these aims:

Part 1 – Dissecting Words to Aid Understanding

In this part, we provide you with prefixes and suffixes that will support you in breaking words down into components in order to aid understanding. Once you become familiar with these prefixes and suffixes, you will start to find that you can interpret terms more readily.

Part 2 – Alphabetic Glossary

This is the main body of the book where we provide an alphabetic glossary listing each term, guidance on its pronunciation and its definition. We have also coded each entry to indicate whether it is normally associated with anatomy and physiology or with pathophysiology.

Part 3 – Notes

Whilst detailed, this book is not exhaustive so space has been left for you to write in your own terms as you encounter and learn them so you can steadily build your vocabulary and deepen your understanding of the biosciences.

PART 1
DISSECTING WORDS TO AID UNDERSTANDING

The terminology associated with anatomy, physiology and pathophysiology can sometimes feel like a foreign language and in essence you would be right; the terms are primarily derived from Greek and Latin. However, a good starting point for learning and understanding the terminology is to break the words down into their separate components of prefix and suffix. Once you have a good working knowledge of those parts, learning and understanding the terms becomes much easier.

It is important to have a good grasp of the terminology as it is used as an international language in healthcare and is necessary for communicating with other members of the interdisciplinary team. Part of being a professional requires you to use the correct terms, remembering that you may have to explain these terms to people in your care.

Prefixes

A prefix appears at the beginning of a word and usually provides a clue as to what to expect in a word's meaning. It generally describes location and intensity. For example, adipo at the beginning of a word usually means it will refer to fat or lipids in some way. Breaking down adipocytes is a good example where *adipo* refers to fat and the suffix (explained below) *cyte* refers to cell - fat cells. A list of commonly used prefixes can be found in Table 1.1.

Suffixes

Suffixes are placed at the end of words to change the original meaning. In terminology associated with anatomy, physiology and pathophysiology, a suffix usually indicates a procedure, condition or disease. In essence, a suffix tells you what is wrong with a specific body part or system or how to fix it. For example, a commonly used suffix is -itis, which means 'inflammation.' When this suffix is paired with the prefix arthro-, meaning joint, the resulting word is arthritis, an inflammation of the joints. A list of commonly used suffixes can be found in Table 1.2.

Table 1.1   Commonly Used Prefixes

Prefix	Meaning
a/an-	Without
ab-	Away from
ad-	Toward, near to
aden(o)	Pertaining to a gland
aer(o)-	Air
adip/o-	Fat
af-	Toward
all(o)-	Other
ana-	Up, apart, backward, again, anew
angi(o)-	Vessel (blood)
ante-	Before, forward
anti-	Against
apo-	Off, away
arteri(o)-	Artery
arthr(o)-	Pertaining to a joint
asthen(o)-	Weakness
ather(o)-	Plaque (fatty substance)

Prefix	Meaning
aut/auto-	Self, own
bar(o)-	Pressure, weight
bas(o)-	Base, opposite of acid
bi-	Two, twice, double
blast(o)-	Germ or cell
brady-	Slow
cardi(o)-	Pertaining to the heart
cata-	Down, lower
cerebr(o)-	Pertaining to the cerebrum
chole-	Pertaining to bile
chondr(o)-	Cartilage
chrom(o)-	Colour
circum-	Around
contra-	Against, counter
cyt(o)-	Pertaining or referring to a cell
de-	Lack of, down, less, removal of
dia-	Through, completely, across, apart
dipl(o)-	Double
dis-	Apart, to separate
dys-	Bad, painful, difficult, abnormal
ecto-	Out, outside
eff-	Out, out of, from
em/en-	In, on
end(o)-	In, within
enter(o)-	Pertaining to the intestines
eosin(o)-	Red, rosy, dawn-coloured
epi-	Above, upon, on
erythr(o)-	Red

Prefix	Meaning
eu-	Good, normal
ex(o)-	Out, away from
extra-	Outside
gastr(o)-	Pertaining to the stomach
glyc(o)-, glycos(o)-	Glucose, sugar
gynaec(o)-	Pertaining to female reproductive organs
haem-	Blood
hapl(o)-	Simple, single
hemi-	Half
hepat(o)-	Liver
hetero-	Other, different
homeo-	Sameness, unchanging, constant
hydr(o)-	Water
hyper-	Above, excessive
hypo-	Deficient, below, under, less than normal
infra-	Beneath
inter-	Between
intra-	Within, into
intro-	Into, within
iso-	Same, equal
juxta-	Near
kary(o)-	Nucleus
kerat(o)-	Hard, horny tissue
kines(o)-, kinesi(o)-	Movement
leuk(o)-	White
lip(o)-	Fat, lipid
ly(o)-	To dissolve, loosen
macro-	Large

Prefix	Meaning
mal-	Bad
medi-	Middle
mega-	Large, enlarged
melan-	Black
meso-	Middle
meta-	Change, beyond
micro-	Small
multi-	Many
my(o)-	Muscle
nas(o)-	Pertaining to the nose
necr(o)-	Death
neo-	New
nephr(o)	Pertaining to the kidney
neur(o)-	Nerve
neutr(o)-	Neutral
noci-	To cause harm, injury or pain
oligo-	Few, less than
oophor(o)-	Pertaining to the ovary
opthalm(o)-	Pertaining to the eye
orchid(o)-	Pertaining to the testicle
oro-	Pertaining to the mouth
oste(o)-	Bone
ot(o)-	Pertaining to the ear
para-	Near, beside, abnormal, apart from, along the side of
patho-	Disease
per-	Through

Prefix	Meaning
peri-	Surrounding, around
phag(o)-	Pertaining to eating, ingesting or engulfing
pharyng(o)-	Pertaining to the pharynx/throat
phleb(o)	Pertaining to veins
pneum(o)-, pneumon(o)-	Lung, air, gas
poly-	Many, much
post-	After, behind
pre-	Before, in front of
pro-	Before, forward
proct(o)-	Pertaining to the rectum
proxim(o)-	Near
pseud(o) -	False
psych(o)-	Pertaining to the mind
pulm(o)-	Pertaining to the lung
pyel(o)-	Pertaining to the kidney
quadri-	Four
retro-	Backward, located behind
rhin(o)-	Pertaining to the nose
sarc(o)-	Flesh (connective tissue)
semi-	Half, partly
somat(o)-	Body
steno-	Narrow, contracted
sub-	Under, below
super-	Above
supra-	Above, upper
syn-/sym-	Together, with
tachy-	Fast, rapid

Prefix	Meaning
tel(o)-	Complete
thorac(o)-	Pertaining to the thorax/chest
thromb(o)-	Clot
trans-	Across, through
tri-	Three, triple
ultra-	Beyond, in excess
vas(o)-	Vessel
viscer(o)-	Internal organs

Table 1.2   Commonly Used Suffixes

Suffix	Meaning
-able, -ible	Ability to, capable of
-aemia, -aemic	Pertaining or referring to blood
-aesthesia	Condition of sensation
-al, -ar	Pertaining to
-algia	Referring to pain
-ary	Pertaining to, connected with
-ase	Enzyme
-ate	Action or state
-blast	Embryonic, immature cell
-centesis	A piercing, pertaining to a procedure in which an organ or body cavity is punctured, often to drain excess fluid or obtain a sample for analysis
-cle, -cula, -cule, -culum, -culus	Diminutive
-crine	To secrete, separate
-cyte	Pertaining or referring to a cell

Suffix	Meaning
-ectasis	Dilation/distension
-ectomy	Removal, cutting out
-emesis	Vomiting
-erg/o	Pertaining or referring to work
-flux	Flow
-form	Shape, structure
-fugal	Movement away from
-genesis, -gen, -genic	Producing, forming
-gram	Record, recording, writing
-ia	State, condition
-ic	Pertaining to
-ile	Pertaining to, characteristic of
-ion	Process, action
-ism	Process, condition
-itis	Inflammation
-ity	State
-kinesis	Movement
-lith	Stone
-logy	Study of/branch of
-lysis	Breakdown, separation, destruction, loosening
-megaly	Enlargement of
-metry	Process of measuring
-oid	Resembling, derived from
-ole	Little, small
-oma	Tumour
-ostomy	Surgical creation of an opening, or hole
-otomy	Surgical incision

Suffix	Meaning
-oxia	Condition of oxygenation
-pathy	Disease or a system for treating disease
-penia	Deficiency of
-phage, -phagia	Eat, swallow, ingestion of, consumption
-phil-	Like, love, attraction to
-phob-	Fear
-plasia	Growth, formation
-plegia	Paralysis of
-pnoea	Pertaining to breathing
-poiesis	Formation
-rrhagia	bleeding from, flow of
-rrhoea	Flow
-sclerosis	Hardening
-sis	State or process
-stasis	To stop, control, place
-tax/o	Order, coordination
-tomy	Cut/incise
-ton/o	Tension
-trophy	Nourishment, development (condition of)
-uria	Refers to urine condition
-zyme	Enzyme

PART 2
ALPHABETIC GLOSSARY

Term	Definition
Abduction *(Ab-duc-shun)*	Movement away from the midline of the body
Abscess *(Ab-ses)*	A collection of pus restricted to a specific area in tissue, organs or confined space
Absorption *(Ab-sorb-shun)*	The process by which one substance absorbs or is absorbed (taken in or assimilated) by another
Absorption (cellular) *(Ab-sorb-shun)*	Movement of nutrients across the intestinal wall into the blood and lymphatic circulation
Acanthosis *(A-can-tho-sis)*	Epidermal hyperplasia (thickening of the skin)
Accommodation	Change in shape of the lens of the eye
Acetylcholinesterase inhibitors *(A-ce-til-col-in-est-er-ase)*	Drugs that inhibit acetylcholinesterase activity (i.e. inhibit the breakdown of acetylcholine)

Key

Primarily associated with anatomy and physiology

Primarily associated with pathophysiology

Term	Definition
Achondroplasia *(A-con-dro-play-see-a)*	A genetic disorder characterised by abnormally slow conversion of cartilage to bone during bone development, resulting in short stature (causing disproportionate body structure: normal size trunk, short limbs)
Acidaemia *(A-sid-e-me-ah)*	The state of low blood pH caused by an increase in hydrogen ions
Acidosis *(A-sid-oh-sis)*	Clinical condition as a result of a low arterial blood pH<7.35. Can be either respiratory or metabolic
Acinar cells *(A-sin-ar)*	Exocrine cells of the pancreas that secrete pancreatic enzymes
Acini *(A-sin-eye)*	Plural of acinus
Acinus *(A-sin-us)*	A respiratory unit made up of alveoli or a small sac-like cavity in a gland, surrounded by secretory cells (berry-like cluster of cells)
Acne vulgaris *(Ack-knee vul-gar-is)*	Chronic inflammatory dermatosis affecting the pilosebaceous unit leading to inflammatory and non-inflammatory lesions
Acquired *(A-kwai-ered)*	Develops after birth (with reference to a condition/disorder)
Acquired Immunodeficiency Syndrome (AIDS)	A syndrome associated with HIV that is characterised by immunosuppression and opportunistic infections, malignant tumours, cachexia and central nervous system (CNS) degeneration
Acromegaly *(A-crow-meg-a-lee)*	Abnormal, large growth of the hands, feet, and face, caused by overproduction of growth hormone by the pituitary gland

Term	Definition
Action potential	The change in electrical potential in the membrane of a neuron to send an electrical impulse along its length
Active transport	The movement of solutes (ions and molecules) across a membrane (usually) against a concentration gradient involving the use of energy (ATP) and carrier proteins
Acute (*A-cute*)	Condition in which signs and symptoms develop suddenly and usually last a short time
Acute kidney injury (AKI)	A rapid decline in kidney function occurring over hours to days, resulting in the inability to maintain fluid, electrolyte and acid-base balances, evidenced by a decrease in glomerular filtration rate and urine output and an increase in nitrogenous waste leading to azotaemia and uraemia
Acute lung injury (ALI)	An acute lung disease with bilateral pulmonary infiltrate consistent with oedema with no evidence of left atrial hypertension
Acute lymphocytic leukaemia (ALL) (*A-cute limb-pho-sit-ick loo-key-me-a*)	Also known as acute lymphoblastic leukaemia, this form of leukaemia arises from lymphoid stem cells. As abnormal cells accumulate in the bone marrow, they crowd out the bone marrow and this prevents the further production of healthy cells

Key

Primarily associated with anatomy and physiology

Primarily associated with pathophysiology

Term	Definition
Acute myeloid leukaemia (AML) (*A-cute my-e-loyd loo-key-me-a*)	An acute form of leukaemia affecting the myeloid stem cells that results in blast cells that do not differentiate into the types of leucocytes needed to fight off pathogens
Acute myocardial Infarction (AMI) (*A-cute my-oh-kar-dee-al in-farc-shun*)	Rupture or erosion of an atherosclerotic plaque with thrombotic occlusion of an epicardial coronary artery and ischaemia across the wall of the heart (myocardium) that leads to infarction (local death of tissue)
Acute on chronic	When someone with a chronic condition has an acute exacerbation of their condition, requiring more intensive treatment
Acute pancreatitis (*A-cute pan-cree-a-tie-tis*)	Reversible inflammation of the pancreas that occurs suddenly due to premature activation of pancreatic enzymes that may be caused by gallstones or increased alcohol intake
Acute respiratory distress syndrome (ARDS)	An acute inflammatory lung injury associated with increased pulmonary vascular permeability, increased lung weight and loss of aerated tissue
Acute tubular necrosis (ATN) (*A-cute chew-bew-lar neh-crow-sis*)	Acute kidney injury (AKI) secondary to damage to the renal tubules as a result of ischaemia and initiation of an inflammatory response that promotes the production of toxic oxygen free radicals leading to oedema, injury and necrosis. The nephrotoxic form is a result of poison, toxins or medication
Adaptive immunity	A specific immune response consisting of antibody responses and cell-mediated responses where each pathogen is 'remembered' by a signature antibody

Term	Definition
Addison's disease	A chronic endocrine disorder in which the adrenal glands do not produce enough steroid hormones due to progressive destruction of the adrenal cortex
Adduction (*A-duck-shun*)	Movement closer to the midline of the body
Adenocarcinoma (*A-den-oh-car-sin-o-ma*)	A tumour formed when glandular cells mutate into cancer cells
Adenoids (tonsils) (*A-den-oids*)	A mass of enlarged lymphatic tissue
Adenoma (*A-den-oh-ma*)	A benign tumour formed from glandular structures in epithelial cells
Adenosine deaminase (ADA) (*A-den-oh-zeen d-am-in-ase*)	An enzyme that eliminates a molecule, called deoxyadenosine, produced when DNA is broken down. ADA converts deoxyadenosine, which is toxic to lymphocytes, to deoxyinosine, which is not toxic
Adenosine triphosphate (ATP) (*A-den-oh-zeen try-foss-fate*)	The energy store of the cell used to power cellular activities
Adenoviruses (*A-den-oh-vi-russ-es*)	Any of a group of DNA viruses discovered in adenoid tissue
Adhesins (*Ad-he-zins*)	Surface molecules that enable bacteria to attach to a host cell
Adhesions (*Ad-he-shuns*)	Fibrous bands of scar tissue that form between tissues

Key

Primarily associated with anatomy and physiology

Primarily associated with pathophysiology

Term	Definition
Adiadochokinesia (*A-die-a-dough-co-kin-e-zee-a*)	Inability to perform rapid alternating movements
Adipocytes (*A-de-po-sites*)	Fat cells that make up adipose tissue
Adipokines (*A-de-po-kins*)	Cell signalling proteins from adipose tissues, a form of cytokine
Adiponectin (*A-de-po-neck-tins*)	A protein hormone involved in regulating glucose levels as well as fatty acid breakdown
Adipose tissue (*A-de-pose tissue*)	Tissue composed of adipocytes, specialist cells that store fat. There are two types; white and brown. Brown adipose tissue is used in infants to generate heat. White adipose tissue is more prevalent in adults and is hormonal, secreting hormones such as leptin that reduces appetite and fat storage
Adjuvant therapy (*A-dew-vant*)	Therapy given in addition to the primary/initial therapy to maximise its effectiveness
Adolescence (*A-dole-s-ants*)	The stage in life when the child turns into an adult (normally between the ages of 10 and 19)
Adrenal (cortical) insufficiency (*A-dreen-al (kor-tick-al)*)	A condition in which the adrenal cortex does not produce adequate amounts of steroid hormones
Adrenocorticotropic hormone (ACTH) (*A-dreen-oh-kor-tick-oh-trow-fic*)	A hormone produced by the pituitary gland that stimulates the production and release of cortisol from the adrenal cortex

Term	Definition
Adrenogenital syndromes (congenital adrenal hyperplasia) (*A-dreen-o-jen-it-al sin-dromes (con-jen-it-al a-dreen-al hi-per-play-see-a)*)	A group of disorders caused by adrenocortical hyperplasia or malignant tumours, leading to abnormal secretion of adrenocortical hormones and characterised by masculinisation of women, feminisation of men, or precocious puberty
Aerobic (*Air-obe-ic*)	Relates to an organism that exists with, or is dependent on, oxygen
Aerobic metabolism (*Air-obe-ic met-a-bo-liz-im*)	Metabolism of glucose in the presence of oxygen
Aetiological epidemiology (*A-tee-oh-lodge-ic-al epp-e-dee-me-ol-oh-gee*)	Searches for factors (hazardous or beneficial) influencing health status (e.g. toxins, poor diet, pathogenic microorganisms, health promoting behaviours)
Agonists (*A-go-nists*)	Substances/drugs which, through binding with receptors, alter cell activity in some way to modify a specific mechanism within the cell; the substance therefore initiates or activates a physiological response when combined with a receptor or a muscle whose action is opposed by another muscle (antagonist)
Agraphia (*A-graf-e-ah*)	Inability to locate the words for writing
Agranulocytes (*A-gran-you-low-sites*)	Leucocytes that have little or no organelles and so do not have a granular appearance

Key

Primarily associated with anatomy and physiology

Primarily associated with pathophysiology

Term	Definition
Akinesia (*a-kin-e-see-ya*)	Impairment of voluntary movement
Albumin (*Al-bew-min*)	The main plasma protein which generates plasma colloidal osmotic pressure and serves as a transport protein
Albuminuria (*Al-bew-min-you-ree-a*)	Presence of albumin in the urine
Aldosterone (*Al-doss-ter-own*)	A hormone produced by the adrenal cortex under the influence of angiotensin II that promotes the reabsorption of sodium in the renal tubule, drawing water with it
Alexia (*a-lex-e-a*)	Reading difficulties
Alkalosis (*Al-ka-low-sis*)	Clinical condition as a result of a high arterial blood pH greater than 7.45. Can be either respiratory or metabolic
Alkaptonuria (*Al-kap-ton-you-ree-a*)	A genetic disorder that prevents the body fully breaking down two amino acids, tyrosine and phenylalanine, leading to build-up of homogenistic acid which may lead to black urine
Alkylating agents (*Al-kill-a-ting*)	The shape of DNA is changed through alkyl forming bonds with the DNA (alkylation) thus inducing cell death or slowing the replication of tumour cells
Allele (*A-leel*)	Alternative form of the same gene located at the corresponding position on homologous chromosomes
Allergen (*Al-er-jen*)	Substance that can cause an allergic reaction
Allergic reaction (*Al-er-jic*)	Type 1 hypersensitivity where a person has a hypersensitive immune response to an environmental substance

Term	Definition
Alloimmunity (*A-low-im-you-nit-e*)	The immune response against the tissue of another individual (e.g. in organ transplantation or blood transfusion)
Alopecia (*A-low-p-sha*)	Hair loss
Alopecia areata (*A-low-p-sha a-ree-at-a*)	A non-cicatricial T cell mediated autoimmune process that targets anagen stage hair follicles, disrupting the growth of hair through destruction of the hair follicle
Alpha-adrenergic receptors (*Al-fa a-dren-er-gic*)	Receptors that, when stimulated by catecholamines, constrict blood vessels, contract uterine muscles, relax intestinal muscles and dilate pupils
Alternative therapy	When a non-mainstream therapeutic intervention is used instead of conventional (Western) medicine
Alveolar ducts (*Al-vee-oh-lar*)	Thin-walled air passages that are subdivisions of bronchioles and lead to alveoli
Alveolar fluid	Fluid lining the alveoli
Alveolar ventilation	The amount of inspired air that reaches the alveoli during a breath
Alveolar ventilation rate	The actual volume of air per minute that reaches the respiratory zone
Alveoli (*Al-vee-oh-lie*)	Small cup-shaped pouches/air sacs at the terminal end of alveolar ducts where gaseous exchange takes place

Key

Primarily associated with anatomy and physiology

Primarily associated with pathophysiology

Term	Definition
Alzheimer's Disease (*Alts-hime-ers*)	A neurodegenerative condition characterised by the development of intracellular neurofibrillary tangles and deposits of extracellular amyloidal (beta) protein leading to plaque formation in the CNS that leads to decreased acetylcholine production
Amenorrhea (*A-men-or-e-a*)	Absence of menstruation
Amino acid (*A-mean-o*)	Organic compounds that combine to form proteins
Amniotic fluid (*Am-knee-ot-ick*)	Fluid within the amniotic sac
Amniotic fluid embolism	When some amniotic fluid enters the maternal circulation and results in a serious reaction which may result in cardiorespiratory collapse and severe bleeding
Amniotic sac	Sac containing amniotic fluid in which the embryo/fetus is surrounded
Amphiarthroses (*Am-fee-ar-thro-seas*)	Joint with limited movement
Ampulla (*Am-pule-a*)	Sac containing hair cells embedded in the cupula
Amygdala (*A-mig-da-la*)	Part of the limbic system of the brain that contributes to storage of emotional experiences as memories and regulates emotional learning
Amylase (*A-me-laze*)	An enzyme that digests carbohydrates
Amyloidosis (*A-me-loid-o-sis*)	A build-up of amyloid protein (an abnormal protein) in organs and tissues impairing their function

Term	Definition
Amyotrophic lateral sclerosis (ALS) (*A-me-o-trow-fic lat-er-al sclair-o-sis*)	*See* Motor neuron disease
Anabolism (*A-na-bo-liz-im*)	The building up or synthesising of large and complex molecules. This process requires energy
Anaemia (*A-knee-me-a*)	Deficiency of erythrocytes or haemoglobin
Anaemic hypoxia (*A-knee-mick hi-pox-e-a*)	When blood is unable to carry enough oxygen to the tissues
Anaerobic (*A-ner-o-bik*)	Relates to an organism that exists without, or is not dependent on, oxygen
Anaesthesia (*A-naz-thee-zee-a*)	The practice of administering medications to block the feeling of pain and other sensations. General anaesthesia also causes unconsciousness
Anaesthetic (*A-naz-thet-ic*)	Drug/agent that blocks nociception or awareness of pain
Anagen phase (*A-na-jen*)	First phase of hair growth
Anal canal	Terminal end of the gastrointestinal tract
Analgesia (*A-nal-gee-zee-a*)	Drug/agent that diminishes nociception without loss of consciousness

Key

Primarily associated with anatomy and physiology

Primarily associated with pathophysiology

Term	Definition
Anaphylactic reaction (*A-na-phil-ack-tic*)	A systemic response to a hypersensitivity reaction (type 1) resulting in life-threatening clinical features such as difficulty in breathing due to severe bronchoconstriction, low blood pressure as a result of vasodilation and widespread oedema
Anaphylactic shock	Extreme allergic hypersensitive reaction to an antigen which can be life-threatening
Anaplasia (*A-na-play-zee-a*)	When cells are poorly differentiated (normally seen in cancer cells)
Androgenic alopecia (*An-dro-jen-ick a-low-p-sha*)	Male pattern baldness – polygenetic hair loss in genetically susceptible hair follicles in androgen-dependent areas of the scalp
Androgens (*An-dro-jens*)	Male sex hormones
Anencephaly (*A-nen-kef-a-lee*)	Neural tube defect in which major portions of the brain, skull and scalp fail to develop
Aneuploidy (*A-new-ploy-dee*)	An abnormal number of chromosomes in a cell (not an exact multiple of the haploid number i.e. 23)
Aneurysm (*A-nur-is-im*)	The ballooning and widening at a specific point of an artery as a result of weakening of the arterial wall
Angina (pectoris) (*An-jai-na*)	Angina, meaning pain, and pectoris, meaning chest, is chest pain. This normally refers to pain incurred as a result of myocardial ischaemia and occurs when myocardial oxygen demands are increased (e.g. during exercise)
Angiogenesis (*An-gee-oh-gen-e-sis*)	The formation of new blood vessels

Term	Definition
Angioplasty (*An-gee-oh-plas-tee*)	An endovascular procedure to widen narrowed or obstructed blood vessels, often through dilation with a balloon. The procedure enables the placement of a stent
Angiotensin converting enzyme (ACE) (*An-gee-oh-ten-sin*)	A hormone produced by the lungs and proximal convoluted tubules in the nephrons of the kidney that converts angiotensin I to angiotensin II
Angiotensin converting enzyme (ACE) inhibitors	Drugs that block the conversion of angiotensin I to angiotensin II (the active form) therefore preventing its effects. Angiotensin II leads to biological responses that increase blood pressure, thus blocking its production will lower blood pressure
Angiotensin I	A biological inactive plasma protein converted to angiotensin II by angiotensin converting enzyme (ACE)
Angiotensin II	A hormone that brings about a number of responses designed to increase blood volume and blood pressure
Angiotensinogen (*An-gee-oh-ten-sin-oh-jen*)	A plasma protein produced by the liver and converted by renin to angiotensin I
Ankylosis (*An-key-low-sis*)	Joint stiffening and immobility due to fusion of the bones
Anomia (*A-know-me-ah*)	Inability to name an object

Key

Primarily associated with anatomy and physiology

Primarily associated with pathophysiology

Term	Definition
Anomic aphasia (*A-nom-ic a-faze-e-ah*)	Persistent inability to supply words for the things the person wants to say
Anorexia (*A-nor-x-e-ah*)	When the normal physiological stimuli that produce hunger remain intact but there is a lack of desire to eat
Anosmia (*A-noz-me-ah*)	Loss of olfaction (smell)
Anovulation (*A-nov-you-lay-shun*)	When ovaries do not release an oocyte during a menstrual cycle
Anoxia (*A-nox-e-ah*)	An extreme form of hypoxia in which there is total depletion of oxygen
Antagonists (*An-tag-on-ists*)	Substances/drugs which interact with a cell receptor and, by so doing, interfere with or inhibit the physiological action of another substance. They therefore inhibit the action of the other substance. *Also* a muscle that opposes an action of another muscle (agonist)
Anterior cord syndrome	Damage to the anterior two thirds of the spinal cord or the anterior spinal artery leading to loss of motor function, pain and temperature sensation below area of injury/damage
Anterolateral pathways (*An-ter-oh-lat-er-al*)	Sensory pathways for temperature, pain and coarse touch sensations to the brain
Anthracycline (*An-thra-cyc-lean*)	A type of drug derived from the bacteria *Streptomyces* used in cancer chemotherapy

Term	Definition
Antibodies (*An-tea-bod-ees*)	Glycoprotein immunoglobulins (Igs), produced by lymphocytes, that combine with antigens to inactivate them by changing the antigen's chemical composition, render them immobile or preventing them from penetrating cells
Antidiuretic hormone (ADH) (*An-tea-die-your-et-ick*)	A hormone produced by the hypothalamus and released by the pituitary gland. It results in water reabsorption in the renal tubule to retain/increase water levels in the body
Antigen (*An-tea-jen*)	Any substance foreign to the body that evokes an immune response
Antigen-Antibody Complexes	Complexes formed by the binding of antibodies to antigens – or immune complexes
Antigen presenting cells	A type of immune cell that enables a T cell to recognise an antigen in order to generate an immune response against the antigen
Antimetabolites (*An-tea-met-ab-oh-lights*)	Substances that disrupt metabolic pathways of the cell and interfere with nucleic acid metabolism thus preventing normal cell division
Antinuclear antibodies (ANA) (*An-tea-new-kle-ar*)	A type of autoantibody that attacks protein structures within the nucleus of a cell. Also known as antinuclear factor (ANF)
Antiretroviral drugs (*An-tea-re-trow-vi-ral*)	Drugs that interfere with the life cycle of a virus and stop its progression

Key

Primarily associated with anatomy and physiology

Primarily associated with pathophysiology

Term	Definition
Anti-tumour antibiotics	Antibiotics that affect the function of DNA by binding to it and preventing normal cell division and function
Anuria (*An-you-ree-ah*)	Complete suppression of urine formation, with no or minimal output
Anus (*A-nus*)	Opening at the terminal end of the gastrointestinal tract through which faeces are eliminated
Aortic stenosis (*A-or-tic sten-o-sis*)	Narrowing of the aorta that restricts the blood flow leaving the left ventricle
Aperture (*A-per-ture*)	Opening, hole or gap
Aphasia (*A-faze-e-ah*)	Severe difficulty or inability with producing or understanding language and/or speech. Usually due to left-sided brain damage. May be unable to speak. Also refers to a group of language disorders
Aplastic anaemia (*A-plas-tic a-knee-me-ah*)	A form of anaemia where there is a failure in the production of the haematopoietic stem cells in the bone marrow
Apneustic centre (*Ap-new-stik*)	Area in the lower pons responsible for regulating ventilation (with the pneumotaxic centre)
Apocrine gland (*Ap-oh-krin*)	Sweat gland with ducts that open into hair follicles rather than directly onto the surface of the skin and produce sweat containing fats and proteins. Specialised apocrine glands produce ear wax (ceruminous glands) and milk (mammary glands)
Apoptosis (*A-pop-toe-sis*)	Programmed cell death

Term	Definition
Appendicitis (*A-pen-de-sigh-tis*)	Inflammation with or without infection of the vermiform appendix
Appendicular skeleton (*A-pen-dik-yu-lar*)	Bones of the arms and legs and those bones that attach them to the axial skeleton
Appendix (vermiform) (*A-pen-dix (verm-e-form)*)	A tube of about 9cm in length attached to the caecum. It contains a large amount of lymphoid tissue
Apraxia (*A-prax-e-ah*)	Lack of awareness of certain body parts and/or surrounding space. Difficulty with motor planning for tasks of movements
Aquaretics (*Ack-wa-ret-iks*)	A class of drug that promotes aquaresis: excretion of water without loss of electrolytes. *See also* Vaptans
Aqueduct stenosis (*A-kwe-duct sten-oh-sis*)	A congenital narrowing of the channel between the third and fourth ventricles of the brain
Arachnoid mater (*A-rak-noid ma-ter*)	Lining of the brain separated from the dura mater by the dural space and from the pia mater below by the subarachnoid space. It contains large blood vessels and arachnoid villi for reabsorption of CSF
Arachnoid villi (*A-rak-noid vill-eye*)	Small projections of the arachnoid matter of the brain that reabsorb CSF
Archaea (*Ar-kay-ah*)	Microorganisms similar to bacteria in size and structure but genetically and functionally dissimilar from them. They often exist in extreme environmental conditions

Key

Primarily associated with anatomy and physiology

Primarily associated with pathophysiology

Term	Definition
Arrector pili (*A-rek-tor pee-lie*)	Smooth muscle fibres attached to hair follicles
Arrhythmias (*A-rith-me-ahs*)	Irregular or abnormal heart rhythms; disorders of the cardiac conduction cycle
Arrhythmogenesis (*A-rith-mo-jen-eh-sis*)	The development or onset of arrhythmia
Arrhythmogenic (*A-rith-mo-jen-ick*)	Producing or tendency to produce cardiac arrhythmias
Arteries (*Art-er-ease*)	Blood vessels that carry blood away from the heart
Arterioles (*Ar-tear-e-oles*)	Small arteries
Arteriosclerosis (*Ar-tear-e-oh-sclair-o-sis*)	When the arterial walls become thickened and hardened as smooth muscle is replaced by collagen and hyaline cartilage. No lipid material is deposited. The blood vessel becomes less compliant and is associated with raised blood pressure
Arthralgia (*Ar-thral-gee-ah*)	Joint pain
Arthritis (*Ar-thry-tis*)	Joint inflammation
Arthus reaction (*Ar-thus*)	A severe, local immune reaction to the intradermal injection of a vaccine into a sensitised host
Articular capsule (*Ar-tik-you-lar*)	A sleeve-like structure that encloses the synovial cavity
Articular cartilage	Thin layer of hyaline cartilage that covers the epiphysis of one bone where it forms a joint with another bone
Articulation (*Ar-tick-you-lay-shun*)	*See* Joint

Term	Definition
Ascending (afferent) neurons (*A-send-ing (af-er-ent)*)	Neurons that carry information up the spinal cord to the brain for processing
Ascites (*A-see-tees*)	Accumulation of fluid in the peritoneal cavity
Asepsis (*A-sep-sis*)	The absence of microorganisms
Asthenozoospermia (*As-then-oh-zoo-sper-me-ah*)	Sperm that have poor motility
Asthma (*Ass-ma*)	*See* bronchial asthma
Astrocytes (*As-tro-sites*)	Neuroglia in the CNS that support surrounding cells, form the blood brain barrier, and regulate the external chemical environment of neurons by removing excess ions and promoting re-uptake of neurotransmitters released during synaptic transmission
Asynergia (*A-sin-er-gee-ah*)	Loss of coordination of motor movements
Atelectasis (*A-tel-eck-ta-sis*)	Lack of gas exchange within alveoli, due to alveolar collapse or fluid consolidation
Atheroma (*A-ther-oh-ma*)	A reversible build-up of degenerative material in the inner layer of an artery wall consisting of macrophages, fats, calcium and fibrous connective tissue

Key

Primarily associated with anatomy and physiology

Primarily associated with pathophysiology

Term	Definition
Atheroprone (*A-ther-oh-prone*)	Prone to development of atherosclerosis
Atherosclerosis (*A-ther-oh-sclair-oh-sis*)	Chronic inflammatory disease where atheroma builds up in the arteries as plaque is laid down and this in time narrows the arteries and reduces the blood flow
Atoms (*A-toms*)	The basic building blocks of matter
Atopy (*A-top-e*)	The genetic tendency to develop allergic diseases such as allergic rhinitis, asthma and atopic dermatitis (eczema) associated with heightened immune responses to common allergens, especially inhaled and food allergens
Atrial fibrillation (AF) (*A-tree-al*)	A disorder with uncoordinated, irregular atrial contractions that result in deterioration of atrial function
Atrial flutter	Organised atrial rhythm with a rate of typically 250–350 beats per minute
Atrial natriuretic peptide (ANP) (*A-tree-al na-truer-et-ick pep-tide*)	A hormone released from the muscle of the atria of the heart when blood volume is increased, promoting the excretion of sodium in the renal tubule, taking water with it
Atrial septal defect (ASD)	Shunting of blood between the systemic and the pulmonary circulations via a patent foramen ovale, a secundum atrial septal defect or atrial shunting effect at atrial level
Atrioventricular (AV) bundle (*A-tree-oh-ven-trick-u-lar*)	Specialised nerve tract that divides into right and left bundle branches which pass down the septum of the heart dividing out to each ventricle to distribute the impulse

Term	Definition
Atrioventricular (AV) node	Specialised autorhythmic cells in the wall of the septum of the heart that delay the impulse temporarily before conducting it down to the ventricles through the atrioventricular bundle
Atrioventricular septal defect (AVSD)	A spectrum of defects where there is incomplete development of the atrioventricular septum alongside atrioventricular (AV) valve abnormalities
Atrioventricular valves	Valves between the atria and ventricles
Atrium (*A-tree-um*)	Upper chamber of the heart, of which there are two, which receive blood into the heart and pump it into the ventricles. The right atrium receives deoxygenated blood from the veins of systemic circulation, the left atrium oxygenated blood from the pulmonary vein
Atrophy (*A-trow-fee*)	When cells decrease in size resulting in wasting of part of the organ or structure of the body
Atypia (*A-tip-e-ah*)	Cells that appear abnormal but are not malignant
Auditory tube	*See* Eustachian tube
Aura (*Or-ah*)	A subjective sensation including experiences of dreamlike feelings, alterations in smells, hearing, vision or other sensation.

Key

Primarily associated with anatomy and physiology

Primarily associated with pathophysiology

Term	Definition
Aura (continued)	This disturbance of perception may represent a focal electrical disturbance
Auricle (pinna) (*Or-ick-ill* or *Or-ick-ul*)	Fleshy part of the ear
Autism spectrum disorder (ASD) (*Awh-tis-im*)	A group of neurodevelopmental disorders with symptoms that are seen on a continuum ranging from mild to severe. These symptoms include deficits in social reciprocity, communication challenges and repetitive behaviours that may be considered by some as unusual and restrictive
Autoantigens	An antigen that, despite belonging to the host, is the target of a humoral or cell-mediated immune response, e.g. as in autoimmune disease
Autoimmune disease (*Awh-toe-ih-mune*)	*See* Autoimmunity
Autocrine (*Awh-toe-krine*)	Relating to a hormone which has an effect only on the cells which produce it
Autoimmunity/ Autoimmune disease	When the immune system fails to recognise self-antigens and reacts to them as (foreign) antigens
Autologous immune enhancement therapy (AIET) (*Awh-toe-low-gus*)	When immune cells from the person's own body are extracted and treated to increase their efficacy against cancer
Autonomic dysreflexia (*Awh-tow-nom-ick*)	A syndrome whereby the sympathetic nervous system is hyperstimulated (e.g. raising blood pressure excessively) but where there is little or no parasympathetic response to counter-balance this sympathetic reflex activity

Term	Definition
Autonomic nervous system	A division of the nervous system that contains cranial and spinal nerves that subconsciously control visceral organs (including those of the circulatory, digestive and respiratory systems) through regulating involuntary activities via its sympathetic and parasympathetic subdivisions
Autoregulation	The inherent ability of an organ to maintain a constant blood flow despite changes in perfusion pressure
Autorhythmic cells (*Awh-toe-rith-mik*)	Cells of the conduction system that initiate and distribute electrical impulses to adjacent cells which stimulate heart muscle to contract
Autosomal aneuploidy (*Awh-toe-zo-mal a-new-ploy-dee*)	When individual autosomal chromosomes are missing or an extra one is present
Autosomal inheritance	A pattern of inheritance in which the transmission of traits depends on the presence or absence of particular alleles on the autosomes
Autosome (*Awh-toe-zome*)	Any chromosome that is not a sex chromosome
Avascular (*A-vas-que-lar*)	Referring to the absence of blood vessels
Axial skeleton (*Ax-e-al*)	The bones of the skull, vertebral column, ribs and sternum which form the central axis of the body and support the head, neck and torso

Key

Primarily associated with anatomy and physiology

Primarily associated with pathophysiology

Term	Definition
Axon (*Ax-on*)	Long projection in a neuron that carries action potentials
Axon terminal	End(s) of an axon
Azoospermia (*A-zoo-sper-me-ah*)	The absence of sperm in semen
Azotaemia (*A-zo-tae-me-ah* or *A-zo-team-e-ah*)	An increased blood serum level of urea, and frequently of creatinine, caused by both renal insufficiency and renal failure
Bacteraemia (*Back-ter-e-me-ah*)	Bacteria in the blood
Bacteria (*Back-tear-e-ah*)	Plural of bacterium – a single-celled spherical, spiral, or rod-shaped microorganism that appears singly or in chains, existing independently or parasitically
Bacteriophages (*Back-tear-e-oh-faa-jes*)	A virus that infects and replicates within a bacterium
Balanitis (*Baa-lan-eye-tis*)	Inflammation of the glans penis
Baroreceptors (*Ba-row-re-cep-tors*)	Sensory receptors that respond to changes in pressure
Basal cells (taste) (*Bay-zal*)	Stem cells located at the periphery of taste buds that mature into taste cells to replace those that have died
Basal ganglia/nuclei (*Bay-zal gang-lee-ah/new-klee-eye*)	Nuclei of grey matter buried within the white matter
Basal metabolic rate	The rate at which energy is used while at rest to maintain vital organ functions
Basal nuclei (*Bay-zal new-klee-eye/gang-lee-ah*)	See Basal ganglia

Term	Definition
Basophils (*Bay-zo-fills*)	Granulocytes that assist in the inflammatory response by secreting histamine and heparin which increases blood flow by vasodilation and thinning the blood
B cells	Lymphocytes that recognise specific antigens and produce antibodies
Becker muscular dystrophy (BMD) (*Dis-tro-fee*)	Similar to Duchenne muscular dystrophy (DMD) but occurs later in childhood with slower, less severe progression
Benign (*Be-nine*)	When neoplasms have well differentiated cells that are encapsulated, and do not metastasise
Benign cystic teratomas (*Be-nine sis-tik ter-a-toe-maz*)	Germ cell tumours derived from all germ cell layers but mainly ectoderm
Benign prostatic hyperplasia (BPH) (*Be-nine pros-ta-tic hi-per-play-see-ah*)	Hyperproliferation of epithelial and stromal cells in the transitional zone of the prostate gland
Beta-adrenergic receptors (*Be-ta a-dren-er-jic*)	Receptors that, when stimulated by catecholamines, increase heart rate, stimulate cardiac contraction, dilate bronchi, dilate blood vessels and relax the uterus

Key

Primarily associated with anatomy and physiology

Primarily associated with pathophysiology

Term	Definition
Beta-blockers	Drugs that are beta-adrenergic blocking agents, preventing other substances from binding with the receptors. This reduces sympathetic nervous system stimulation of the cardiovascular system, lowering blood pressure
Bile	Liquid produced by the liver containing water, salts, mucus, cholesterol, lecithin and bilirubin that is then stored and concentrated in the gallbladder. It's function is to aid the digestion of lipids
Bilirubin (*Bill-ih-rube-in*)	A breakdown product of haemoglobin converted from biliverdin
Biliverdin (*Bill-ih-ver-din*)	An intermediate substance produced in the degradation of haemoglobin that is converted to bilirubin
Binge eating disorder	A condition in which a person feels compelled to eat in large quantities on a frequent basis, regardless of their state of hunger. This is often followed by feelings of guilt, disgust and low mood
Bioavailability	The amount/proportion of an administered dose of unchanged drug that reaches the systemic circulation and therefore is available to act on its target
Biofilms	Complex multicellular masses consisting of interactive bacterial cells attached to a solid surface or to each other
Bipolar disorder	Enduring mood disorder whereby the person experiences periods of mania and hypomania alternating with periods of depression
Blastocyst (*Blas-toe-sist*)	Structure formed in early pregnancy by development of a solid ball of cells (the morula) which develops a fluid filled space and then imbeds into the uterine wall at about day seven of pregnancy

Term	Definition
Blood	Part of the extracellular fluid (ECF) contained within blood vessels that consists of plasma and blood cells
Blood brain barrier (BBB)	A structural and chemical barrier that strictly regulates substances passing from the circulatory system into the nervous system
Blood pressure	The pressure exerted by the blood against the arterial walls by the pumping force of the heart = cardiac output X peripheral resistance
Blood vessels	The tubes forming the circulation through which the blood is transported around the body. Arteries carry blood away from the heart, veins carry blood back to the heart and the fine capillaries join the two and permit the fluid in the blood to enter the ECF surrounding the cells
B-lymphocyte (*Bee limph-oh-site*)	Type of lymphocyte that differentiates into plasma cells that synthesise antibodies to react with specific antigens that stimulate them
Bolus (*Bow-lus*)	A small rounded mass of a substance (e.g. chewed food)
Bone remodelling	Process where old bone is replaced with new bone (taking approximately 160–200 days)
Borborygmus (*Bore-bor-ig-mus*)	Rumbling sound made by movement of intestinal fluid/gas

Key

Primarily associated with anatomy and physiology

Primarily associated with pathophysiology

Term	Definition
Bowman's capsule	A cup-shaped sac at the beginning of a nephron that collects filtrate from the glomerulus which it encloses
Brachial plexus (*Bray-key-al pleck-sus*)	A group of neurons extending to the arms
Bradycardia (*Brad-e-car-dee-ah*)	Slow heart rate, usually less than 60 beats per minute
Bradykinesia (*Brad-e-kin-e-ze-ah*)	Slowness of movement possibly with weakness, tremor and rigidity
Bradykinin (*Brad-e-ki-nin*)	An inflammatory mediator that causes contraction of smooth muscle and dilation of blood vessels
Bradypnoea (*Brad-e-knee-ah*)	Decreased respiratory rate
Brain tissue oxygenation (PbtO$_2$)	Partial pressure of oxygen in the brain tissue
Broad spectrum antibiotics	Antibiotics that act against both gram-positive and gram-negative bacteria
Broca's aphasia	Non-fluent aphasia – severely reduced speech output as Broca's area of the brain has been affected. Speech is limited mainly to short utterances of less than four words with limited access to vocabulary. Formation of sounds is laborious and clumsy but the person may understand speech and be able to read, but have limited writing ability
Bronchi (*Bron-kai*)	The divisions of the trachea at the inferior end

Term	Definition
Bronchial asthma (*Bron-key-al ass-ma*)	A chronic inflammatory disease, commonly known as asthma, associated with the release of inflammatory mediators from mast cells in the airways leading to a response clinically manifested as expiratory wheeze, experience of chest tightness, dyspnoea, tachypnoea and cough
Bronchial tree	A highly branched system of air conducting passages that extends from the primary bronchus to the terminal bronchioles
Bronchiectasis (*Bron-key-eck-ta-sis*)	The permanent dilation of the bronchi caused by destruction of the bronchial wall and elastic supporting tissue
Bronchioles (*Bron-key-oles*)	Small continuations of the airway, derived from bronchi
Bronchiolitis (*Bron-key-oh-lie-tis*)	The most common lower respiratory tract infection in the first year of life; it is caused by a range of viruses
Bronchoconstriction (*Bron-co-con-stric-shun*)	Constriction of the airways in the lungs as a result of contraction of surrounding smooth muscle
Bronchospasm (*Bron-co-spa-zim*)	Spasm of bronchial smooth muscle resulting in narrowing of the bronchi
Brown-Séquard syndrome (lateral cord syndrome) (*Brown see-kar sin-drome*)	Spinal cord injury with ipsilateral (belonging to or occurring on the same side of the body) muscle paralysis (corticospinal tract injury), ipsilateral loss of vibration and position sensation (posterior column injury)

Key

Primarily associated with anatomy and physiology

Primarily associated with pathophysiology

Term	Definition
Brudzinski sign (*Brood-zin-ski*)	Flexion of the knees and hips when the neck is flexed forward rapidly
B-type natriuretic peptide (BNP) (*Na-tree-ur-et-ick peptide*)	A polypeptide released by the ventricles of the heart in response to excessive stretching of the heart or heart failure
Buccal mucosa (*Bew-kal mew-co-sa* or *Bu-kal mew-co-sa*)	Mucosa of the buccal cavity (mouth)
Budd-Chiari syndrome (*Bud key-ar-ee*)	Obstruction of the hepatic vein draining the liver
Bulbar stricture (*Bul-bar*)	Stricture in the bulbar urethra which can reduce urine flow
Bulbourethral glands (*Bul-bo-you-re-thral*)	Glands that produce 10% of seminal fluid
Bullae (*Bew-lay*)	Large air spaces formed from the destruction of alveoli in emphysema
Bullous (*Bull-us*)	Characterised by blisters
Bundle of His	*See* Atrioventricular bundle
Butterfly fracture	Fracture where two oblique fracture lines meet to form a wedge-shaped fracture resembling a butterfly
Cachexia (*Ca-check-see-ah* or *Ca-ceck-see-ah*)	Weight loss, muscle atrophy, fatigue and weakness caused by the release of inflammatory cytokines, loss of appetite and high metabolic rate. It is characterised by physical wasting
Caecum (*See-kum*)	First part of the large intestine
Calcification (*Kal-sif-ih-kay-shun*)	Accumulation of calcium salts in a body tissue
Calibre (*Kal-ih-bur*)	Internal diameter

Term	Definition
Callus (*Kal-us*)	Bony healing tissue formed around the ends of a fracture
Calyces (*Kal-ih-sees*)	Chambers of the kidney through which urine passes
Cancer	A disease of the cell, where abnormal cell growth and division is uncontrolled, leading to altered function of cells and tissue
Capillaries (*Ka-pill-ar-ease*)	Small blood vessels that link arterioles to venules and enable exchange of water, nutrients and waste products between the blood and the tissues
Carbohydrates (*Kar-bo-hi-drates*)	Macronutrients that are a key source of energy for the body
Carboxypeptidase (*Kar-box-e-pep-tid-ase*)	An enzyme that digests proteins
Carcinogenesis (*Kar-sin-oh-jen-ih-sis*)	When a normal cell is changed into a malignant cell through changes in its genetic structure
Carcinogenic (*Kar-sin-oh-jen-ick*)	Any substance that can induce carcinogenesis
Carcinogens (*Kar-sin-oh-jens*)	Substances capable of inducing cancer
Carcinoma (*Kar-sin-oh-ma*)	Cancer that originates in the epithelial tissue of the skin or tissue that lines the internal organs

Key

Primarily associated with anatomy and physiology

Primarily associated with pathophysiology

Term	Definition
Cardiac cycle	One complete heartbeat during which the heart contracts (systole) and relaxes (diastole)
Cardiac output	The volume of blood pumped out of the heart per minute = stroke volume X heart rate
Cardiac tamponade (*Tam-po-nad*)	Fluid in the pericardium compressing the heart
Cardiogenic shock (*Kar-dee-oh-jen-ick*)	A type of shock that occurs because the heart is no longer able to pump blood round the body adequately
Cardiomyopathies (*Kar-dee-oh-my-op-a-thees*)	A group of cardiac disorders that affect the myocardium
Cardiomyopathy (*Kar-dee-oh-my-op-a-thee*)	Disease of the heart muscle which affects its size, shape and structure, often including hypertrophy
Cardiovascular disease	Diseases that affect the heart or blood vessels. See coronary artery disease
Carpal bones (*Kar-pal*)	Eight small bones of the wrist
Carrier proteins	*See* Transport proteins
Cartilage (*Kar-till-idge*)	A strong, flexible and semi-rigid connective tissue
Cartilaginous joint (*Kar-till-ag-in-us*)	Type of joints connected by cartilaginous material
Catabolism (*Ka-tab-oh-lism*)	The breaking down of nutrients to provide energy and raw materials for anabolism
Catagen phase (*Kat-a-jen*)	Second phase of hair growth
Catalyst (*Kat-a-list*)	A substance that accelerates chemical reactions without themselves being used up

Term	Definition
Catecholamines (*Kat-eh-kol-a-meens*)	Hormones/neurotransmitters (such as dopamine, noradrenaline (norepinephrine), and adrenaline (epinephrine)) produced by the adrenal glands, the brain and some specialised nerve cells that stimulate alpha-adrenergic and beta-adrenergic receptors
Cauda equina (*Kaw-da eh-kwine-ah*)	Nerves resembling a horse's tail that extend from the lower spinal cord down to the sacrum and supply the pelvic organs and lower limbs
Cauda equina syndrome	Syndrome where there is compression of the lumbar, sacral and coccygeal nerve roots extending from the conus medullaris affecting innervation of legs, feet and pelvic organs
Caudal neuropore (*Kaw-dal neu-row-pore*)	Temporary opening at the extreme caudal end of the neural tube
Cell differentiation	The process by which a less specialised cell becomes more specialised
Cell-mediated immunity	The immune response to an antigen involving the activation of phagocytes, antigen-specific cytotoxic T cells, and the release of cytokines

Key

Primarily associated with anatomy and physiology

Primarily associated with pathophysiology

Term	Definition
Cell/plasma membrane	Double layered lipid membrane including proteins that control movement of substances into and out of the cell thus determining composition of cytoplasm (cell contents excluding organelles, largely ions, water and nutrients)
Cellular respiration	Metabolic processes that occur in cells to create energy and waste from nutrients
Central cord syndrome	Spinal cord injury with disproportionately greater motor impairment in arms than legs and accompanying bladder dysfunction. Anteroposterior compressive forces distribute pressure and damage onto the corticospinal tracts innervating the arms
Central nervous system (CNS)	The division of the nervous system made up of the brain and spinal cord
Central neurogenic diabetes insipidus (CNDI) (*Neu-ro-jen-ick die-a-bee-tees in-sip-id-us*)	A condition where there is a deficit in the production and secretion of ADH as a result of injury or genetic defect to the neurohypophysis and therefore there is insufficient amounts to stimulate the renal tubule to reabsorb water and concentrate the urine
Central pontine myelinolysis (*Pon-tine my-e-lin-ol-ih-sis*)	An irreversible demyelination of neurons in the pons which occurs from too rapid serum sodium level correction
Central precocious puberty (*Pre-co-shus*)	The early activation of the hypothalamic-pituitary-gonadal axis that triggers early puberty
Centriacinar (*Sen-tree-a-sin-ar*)	Refers to the central or proximal parts of the acini

Term	Definition
Centrioles (*Sen-tree-oles*)	Two cylinders in the centrosome at right angles to each other
Centrosome (*Sen-tro-zome*)	Core of the cell cytoskeleton from which single filaments radiate and enable movement of vesicles and organelles
Cerebellar hypoplasia (*Ser-eh-bell-ar hi-po-play-see-ah*)	An incomplete or underdeveloped cerebellum
Cerebellomedullary cistern (*Ser-eh-bell-oh me-dull-ar-e sis-turn*)	CSF filled space that links the ventricles with the subarachnoid space
Cerebellum (*Ser-eh-bell-um*)	Part of the brain that coordinates the muscles of the body, regulates muscle tone and posture, and has an important role in cognition
Cerebral aqueduct (*Ser-e-bral ah-que-duct*)	Connection between the third ventricle and the fourth ventricle
Cerebral contusions	Bruising to cerebral parenchyma, largely due to blunt trauma to the head causing microhaemorrhages
Cerebral lacerations	Tears to the brain tissue
Cerebral oedema (*Ser-e-bral o-dee-ma*)	An increased accumulation of water in the intracellular and interstitial fluids within the brain
Cerebral palsy (*Ser-e-bral paul-zee*)	A group of non-progressive disorders of movement, posture and coordination, occurring in early childhood

Key

Primarily associated with anatomy and physiology

Primarily associated with pathophysiology

Term	Definition
Cerebral perfusion pressure (CPP)	The net pressure gradient that causes cerebral blood to perfuse the tissues of the brain; CPP = MAP (mean arterial pressure) – ICP (Intracranial Pressure)
Cerebral salt wasting syndrome (CSWS)	A condition in which there is a loss of both sodium and water from the ECF as a result of a renal loss of sodium which takes water with it. ADH levels are often elevated in an attempt to reabsorb water. However, the primary cause of water depletion is sodium excretion, which is why it is called a salt wasting syndrome
Cerebrospinal fluid (CSF) (*Se-re-bro-spy-nal*)	Fluid formed in the choroid plexus that protects and nourishes the CNS
Cerebrum (*Se-re-brum*)	Part of the brain consisting of the cerebral cortex (grey matter), underlying white matter, the basal nuclei and the limbic system
Cervix (*Ser-vix*)	Thickened ring of muscle and fibrous tissue at the base of the uterus with a central passage
Chelation therapy (*Chi-lay-shun*)	The use of drugs/infusions that bind iron with a substance that then can be excreted from the body, reducing iron levels in the body
Chemical gastropathy (*Gas-trop-ath-e*)	The injury caused to gastric mucosa from long-term reflux into the stomach of duodenal contents, pancreatic secretions and bile
Chemical senses	The sensations of smell (olfaction) and taste (gustation)
Chemokine (*Key-mo-kyne*)	Signalling cytokine

Term	Definition
Chemokine receptor	Cell membrane protein receptors for chemokines
Chemoreceptors (*Key-mo-re-cep-tors*)	Sensory receptors that respond to changes in the concentration of chemicals
Chemotaxis (*Key-mo-tax-is*)	The chemical attraction of a cell to a location
Chemotherapy (*Key-mo-ther-a-pee*)	The use of drugs to treat cancer: it can be used alone or in combination with other therapies and other anti-cancer drugs. Most chemotherapeutic agents are cytotoxic and act on a specific phase of the cell cycle (cell division)
Chiari malformation (*Key-ar-e*)	When the cerebellar tonsils descend into the foramen magnum, impairing CSF circulation and affect cerebellar function
Chitin (*Kai-tin*)	A fibrous polysaccharide sugar found in the cell walls of fungi
Chlamydia (*Cla-mid-e-a*)	Sexually transmitted infection caused by the bacteria *Chlamydia trachomatis*, a gram–negative obligate intracellular pathogen
Cholangitis (*Kol-an-gi-tis*)	Inflammation of the common bile duct
Cholecystitis (*Ko-le-sis-tie-tis*)	Diffuse inflammation of the gallbladder
Choledocholithiasis (*Ko-ledo-ko-li-thigh-a-sis*)	Gall stones in the common bile duct

Key

Primarily associated with anatomy and physiology

Primarily associated with pathophysiology

Term	Definition
Cholelithiasis (*Ko-lee-li-thigh-a-sis*)	Formation of gall stones through solidification of substances found in bile, primarily cholesterol and bilirubin
Cholesterol (*Ko-les-ter-ol*)	Most common steroid molecule and is the precursor for the steroid hormones
Chondroblasts (*Con-dro-blasts*)	Cells actively producing the components of the extracellular matrix. They may differentiate into chondrocytes
Chondrocytes (*Con-dro-sites*)	Mature cartilage cells derived from chondroblasts
Choriocarcinoma (*Ko-re-o-car-sin-oma*)	A malignant uterine tumour that originates in the fetal chorion
Chorion (*Ko-re-on*)	The outermost membrane surrounding an embryo that contributes to the formation of the placenta
Choroid (*Ko-royd*)	Heavily pigmented layer of the eye that sits behind the retina, nourishing it and preventing light scattering within the eye
Choroid plexus (*Ko-royd plec-sus*)	A network of blood vessels in each ventricle of the brain that produce CSF
Chromatids (*Crow-mat-ids*)	Duplicated chromosomes formed during cell division
Chromosomal abnormality (*Crow-ma-so-mal*)	A disorder that results from a change in the number or structure of chromosomes
Chromosome (*Crow-ma-zome*)	Structures in the nucleus composed of DNA tightly coiled many times around proteins. They are responsible for genetic expression
Chronic (*Kron-ick*)	Persisting for a long time or constantly recurring

Term	Definition
Chronic bronchitis	An inflammatory respiratory condition characterised by a persistent cough and sputum production for at least three months per year for two consecutive years
Chronic illness	An illness that persists over an extended period of time described in terms of months and years rather than days and weeks, and usually longer than three months. The illness may also be progressive
Chronic kidney disease (CKD)	A slow, progressive and irreversible permanent loss of nephrons, tubular absorptive capacity, decline in renal function and loss of endocrine functions. GFR decreases to less than 60 ml/min per 1.73 m^2, albuminuria occurs or both for three or more months
Chronic lymphocytic leukaemia (CLL) (*Lim-fo-sit-ik lu-key-me-a*)	A malignant disorder that originates with lymphoid stem cells and results in immature lymphocytes. It is more common in western society. The cause is largely unknown and it occurs more commonly in those over 50 years of age
Chronic myeloid leukaemia (CML) (*My-ih-loyd lu-key-me-a*)	A chronic form of leukaemia affecting myeloid stem cells. CML is associated with an abnormal chromosome known as the Philadelphia chromosome, affecting chromosomes 22 and 9. In this form of leukaemia, there is an over production of granulocytes and their precursors

Key

Primarily associated with anatomy and physiology

Primarily associated with pathophysiology

Term	Definition
Chronic obstructive pulmonary disease (COPD)	A group of respiratory disorders that are characterised by persistent respiratory symptoms and airflow limitation due to abnormalities caused by exposure to noxious particles or gases
Chronic pancreatitis (*Pan-cre-a-tie-tis*)	The progressive and irreversible fibrotic destruction of the exocrine pancreas that over time leads to the destruction of the endocrine pancreas
Chyle (*Kai-l or Chai-l*)	Collection of chylomicrons in lacteals
Chylomicrons (*Kai-low-my-crons or Chai-low-my-crons*)	Type of lipoprotein created in the small intestine to aid absorption
Chylothorax (*Kai-low-tho-racks or Chai-low-tho-racks*)	The presence of lymphatic fluid in the pleural space
Chyme (*Kaim or Chaim*)	Partly digested food mixed with digestive enzymes
Chymotrypsin (*Kai-mo-trip-sin*)	A digestive enzyme which breaks down proteins in the small intestine
Chymotrypsinogen (*Kai-mo-trip-sin-o-gen or Chai-mo-trip-sin-o-gen*)	A proteolytic enzyme and a precursor of the digestive enzyme chymotrypsin. Formed in the pancreas
Cicatricial (*Sick-a-trish-al*)	Scarring
Cicatricial alopecia (*Sick-a-trish-al a-low-p-sha*)	A form of hair loss where there is progressive and permanent destruction of hair follicles that is followed by replacement with fibrous tissue

Term	Definition
Cilia (*Sil-e-ah*)	Fine hair-like projections from certain cells that sweep in unison to move particles and mucus away
Ciliary body (*Sil-e-ar-e*)	A continuation of the choroid of the eye containing the ciliary muscle and ciliary processes
Ciliary muscle (*Sil-e-ar-e*)	Muscle that encircles the lens of the eye to change its shape to focus the light for vision
Ciliary processes (*Sil-e-ar-e*)	Part of the ciliary body that secretes aqueous humour
Cingulate gyrus/cortex (*Sin-gu-late gi-rus*)	Part of the limbic system thought to integrate emotion and sensory experiences, plus learning and memory
Circadian rhythm (*Sir-kay-de-an*)	The inherent biological clock related to biological processes that occur regularly at about 24-hour intervals
Circumduction (*Sir-cum-duck-shun*)	A combination of flexion, extension, abduction and adduction
Cirrhosis (*Sir-oh-sis*)	An irreversible, inflammatory, fibrotic liver disease in which hepatocytes are destroyed faster than they can be regenerated. Liver tissue becomes scarred and destroyed through inflammation and fibrosis
Citrullination (*Si-trul-in-a-shun*)	The modification of the amino acid arginine to citrulline, a non-essential acid amino
Clavicle (*Cla-vi-kul*)	The collarbone

Key

Primarily associated with anatomy and physiology

Primarily associated with pathophysiology

Term	Definition
Clinical epidemiology (*Ep-e-de-me-ol-oh-gee*)	Describes natural course of a disease in a population and evaluates effects of diagnostic procedures and treatment
Clinical trial	Study in which one group of people with a particular condition receive a specified treatment and their progress is compared with a second control group who are not receiving the active intervention
Clitoris (*Kli-tor-is*)	Female equivalent of the penis in men, containing erectile tissue and responds to sexual arousal by enlarging and becoming firm
Clonic (*Klon-ick*)	Phase of a seizure in which there are violent muscular contractions
Clonus (*Klo-nus*)	Involuntary rhythmic contractions triggered by stretch of the muscle
Cluster headache	Clusters of episodic headaches occurring 1-8 times daily for weeks or months
Coagulation (*Ko-ag-u-lay-shun*)	A complex series of reactions in which positive feedback mechanisms result in blood clot formation
Coarctation of the aorta (CoA) (*Ko-arc-tae-shun*)	A localised narrowing of the aortic lumen secondary to medial wall thickening and infolding aortic wall tissue
Cochlea (*Cock-lee-ah*)	Spiral cavity of the inner ear containing the organ of Corti
Codon (*Ko-don*)	A triplet of nucleotides in the mRNA chain that codes for a specific amino acid in the synthesis of a protein molecule
Coeliac disease (*Sea-lee-ack*)	A condition in which there is malabsorption in the small intestine with associated inflammation

Term	Definition
Cognition (*Cog-nish-un*)	The mental process of acquiring and interpreting knowledge, including perception, intuition, and reasoning
Collagen (*Kol-a-gen*)	The primary structural protein in connective tissue
Collagenase (*Kol-a-gen-aze*)	An enzyme that breaks down collagen
Collateral (*Ko-lat-er-al*)	Secondary or accessory rather than direct or immediate, or a small branch e.g. nerve or blood vessels
Collecting duct	Duct that collects the filtrate from a number of nephrons
Colon (*Ko-lon*)	Largest section of the large intestine between the caecum and the rectum
Colonisation	To become established in a new environment
Colostrum (*Ko-loss-trum*)	First secretion of breast milk after delivery of the baby which contains more white cells and antibodies (particularly IgA) than mature milk (final stage of breast milk)
Colour agnosia (*Ag-nose-e-ah*)	Difficulty identifying colour
Coma (*Ko-ma*)	A state of unconsciousness where the person cannot be aroused and there is no detectable behavioural awareness
Combined immunodeficiency	Impairment of T lymphocyte and/or B lymphocyte development
Commensal (*Ko-men-sal*)	Normal symbiotic flora living on or within the body, deriving benefit without harming or benefiting the host

Key

Primarily associated with anatomy and physiology

Primarily associated with pathophysiology

Term	Definition
Comminuted fracture (*Kom-in-you-tid*)	Fracture of a bone into more than two pieces
Communicable disorders/disease	Disease spread by contact, e.g. by pathogens transmitted to people from other people, from animals (zoonoses), or from other reservoirs of infection in the environment
Community trial	Study examining the effect of an intervention on a community as the unit of study, not individuals
Compact bone	Strong, dense bone tissue
Complement proteins	Plasma proteins that facilitate phagocytosis of bacteria through opsonisation
Complement system	A second major system within innate immunity consisting of a large number (20+) of plasma proteins that facilitate phagocytosis of bacteria through opsonisation
Complementary and alternative medicine	Therapies outside mainstream medicine (i.e. medical approaches to care which originated in Western civilisation)
Complementary therapy	When a non-mainstream therapeutic intervention is used together with conventional (Western) medicine
Compounds	Chemicals made from atoms of different elements joined by chemical bonds
Compression fracture	Fracture where two bones are crushed together through compressive forces
Concentric lamellae (*Kon-sen-trick lam-e-lay*)	Plates of compact bone

Term	Definition
Conchae (*Kon-kay*)	Long, narrow curled shelves of bone
Concussion	When the brain is exposed to rapid acceleration, deceleration, and rotational forces that stretch and distort neural structures, causing transient neurological dysfunction, e.g. headaches and problems with concentration, memory, balance and coordination
Conducting zone	Parts of the airway that deliver inhaled and exhaled air to and from the lungs but in which no gaseous exchange takes place
Conduction	Heat loss as a result of contact with a surface colder than the body
Cones	Photoreceptors sensitive to blue, green and red light. They allow colour vision and are important in day vision
Congenital	Present from birth (with reference to a condition/disorder)
Congenital adrenal hyperplasia	*See* Adrenogenital syndromes
Congenital hypogonadotropic hypogonadism (CHH) (*Hi-po-go-nah-do-tro-pick hi-po-go-na-diz-im*)	A heterogeneous disease characterised by a lack of puberty and infertility secondary to deficient secretion or action of gonadotropin-releasing hormone (GnRH)

Key

Primarily associated with anatomy and physiology

Primarily associated with pathophysiology

Term	Definition
Congestive heart failure	*See* Heart failure
Coning	When intracranial pressure reaches the point of irreversible decompensation, the brain will begin to herniate, forcing the brain to displace into any available space, often through the foramen magnum
Conjunctiva (*Kon-junk-tie-va*)	A thin, transparent protective membrane that coats the anterior surface of the eye, except for the cornea, and the inner surface of the eyelid
Conjunctivitis (*Kon-junk-tiv-eye-tis*)	Inflammation of the conjunctiva of the eye
Connective tissue	Structural tissues that provide structural support for the organs of the body
Consciousness (*Kon-shus-ness*)	A state of explicit awareness dependent on both biological arousal in the brain and the processing of experiences (perception)
Consolidation (pulmonary) (*Kon-sol-id-a-shun*)	When an aerated section of the lung becomes filled with fluid
Constipation	Infrequent or difficult defaecation and usually indicates a decrease in the number of bowel movements per week and hard stools that are difficult to pass
Constriction	Narrowing of the pupil
Contrecoup (*Kon-tre-koo*)	In head injury, damage on the opposite side of the brain from the impact

Term	Definition
Contusion (*Kon-tu-shun*)	A bruise resulting from direct trauma whereby the injured tissues undergo a sequence of events including microscopic rupture of blood vessels, damage to muscle cells, swelling and inflammation
Conus medullaris (*Ko-nuz med-you-lar-is*)	Narrowing of the lumbar part of the spinal cord into a conical shape
Conus medullaris Syndrome	Trauma to the conus medullaris that leads to radicular pain (down the course of the nerve root), bowel and bladder dysfunction, loss of sensation and lower limb weakness relative to the lumbar and sacral nerve pathways affected
Convalescence	The period of recuperation and recovery from disease
Convection (*Kon-vec-shun*)	Heat loss from air being heated as it passes over the body, rises and is replaced by cool air
Convulsion	Overt, major motor manifestations of a seizure
Cor pulmonale (*Kor pull-mon-ah-ley*)	Enlargement of the right side of the heart secondary to lungs or pulmonary blood vessel disease
Core body temperature	The temperature centrally within the body – how warm the vital organs are
Corneocytes (*Kor-knee-oh-sites*)	Terminally differentiated keratinocytes composing most of the stratum corneum, the outermost part of the epidermis

Key

Primarily associated with anatomy and physiology

Primarily associated with pathophysiology

Term	Definition
Coronary artery disease (CAD)	When the major blood vessels that supply the heart with blood, oxygen and nutrients (coronary arteries) become damaged or diseased. Plaque develops over time and reduces myocardial blood flow
Coronary circulation	Blood supply to the heart
Coronary heart disease	*See* Coronary artery disease
Corpus callosum (*Kor-pus kal-oh-sum*)	Major tract of nerve fibres joining the two sides of the brain
Corpus luteum (*Kor-pus loo-tay-um*)	A temporary endocrine structure developed from the follicle after ovulation that secretes fairly high levels of progesterone and medium levels of oestrogen and inhibin
Corpus spongiosum (*Kor-pus spon-gee-oh-sum*)	Cylindrical body of erectile tissue in the penis
Corticospinal tracts (*Kor-te-ko-spy-nal*)	Carries information from the cerebral cortex to the spinal cord
Corticosteroids (*Kor-te-ko-ster-oids*)	Steroid hormones produced in the adrenal cortex (glucocorticoids and mineralocorticoids) that are involved in metabolism and inflammatory response
Cortisol (*Kor-ti-sol*)	A steroid hormone (glucocorticoid class)
Coryzal illness (*Kor-eye-zal*)	Inflammation of nasal cavities, mouth and throat, caused by a virus
Cough (*Kof*)	Protective reflex that helps clear the airways
(Acute) cough (*A-kewt kof*)	A cough that occurs in response to illness that lasts less than 3 weeks

Term	Definition
Chronic cough (*Kron-ick kof*)	A cough that occurs in response to illness and lasts more than 8 weeks. May also be referred to as persistent
Counter anti-inflammatory response syndrome (CARS)	A systemic deactivation of the immune system with the aim of restoring homeostasis from an inflammatory state
Coup (*Koo*)	Under the area of impact in head injury. *See* also Contrecoup
Cranial nerves (*Kray-knee-al*)	Twelve pairs of nerves that extend to the periphery of the body directly from the brain through openings in the skull
C-reactive protein (CRP)	A plasma protein which increases in level in response to inflammation
Creatinine (*Kree-a-tin-een*)	A compound molecule generated from creatine during muscle metabolism
Creatinine clearance	The rate at which creatinine is cleared from the blood by the kidney
Crepitus (*Krep-it-us*)	Grating, crackling or popping sounds or sensations due to air in the subcutaneous tissue, or in damaged bones or joints
Cribriform foramina (*Krib-re-form for-ah-mine-ah*)	Pores in the ethmoid bone of the skull that allow the axon of olfactory neurons to pass through to the olfactory bulb

Key

Primarily associated with anatomy and physiology

Primarily associated with pathophysiology

Term	Definition
Crohn's disease (*Crow-ns*)	A recurrent granulomatous type of inflammatory response that can affect any part of the GIT from the mouth to anus. It is slowly progressive and can be a life-limiting and disabling disease
Croup (*Kroop (sounds like group)*)	An inflammatory condition that affects the airways of babies and young children aged between three months and three years
Cryptorchidism (*Kript-or-kid-ism*)	Undescended testis or testes
Crystallisation (*Kris-tal-eye-zay-shun*)	The formation of crystals
Crystalloid solution (*Kris-ta-loyd*)	The most commonly used type of intravenous fluids; a solution in which crystals can or may form but can diffuse across cell membranes
CT	Computerised tomography (CT), or computerised axial tomography (CAT) – a scan that creates a digital image of structures inside the body from a series of x-rays (ionising radiation)
Cupula (*Kup-you-la*)	A gelatinous membrane in the ampulla
Curettage (*Cure-eh-tage*)	The use of a curette (scoop) to remove uterine tissue
Cushing's syndrome (hypercorticalism) (*Kush-ings sin-drome (Hi-per-kor-tic-al-ism)*)	A metabolic disorder caused by overproduction of corticosteroid hormones by the adrenal cortex
Cyanosis (*Sigh-an-oh-sis*)	Bluish discolouration of skin and/or mucous membranes due to increased levels of deoxygenated blood in the small vessels

Term	Definition
Cyclin-dependent kinases (*Sigh-klin dependent kin-azes*)	Enzymes that bind with cyclins to monitor and control different stages of the cell cycle including repair of DNA at the checkpoints
Cyclins (*Sigh-klins*)	Proteins that control stimulation and progression through the cell cycle
Cystadenomas (*Sist-a-den-oh-maz*)	A benign tumour that develops from ovarian tissue
Cystic fibrosis (CF) (*Sis-tic fi-bro-sis*)	An autosomal recessive condition that occurs owing to mutations in the CFTR (cystic fibrosis transmembrane conductance regulator) gene, resulting in disruption in the transport of salt and water across cell membranes in pancreas, lungs, liver and salivary glands
Cystitis (*Sis-tie-tis*)	Infection/inflammation of the lower urinary tract, primarily the bladder
Cystocele (*Sis-toe-seal*)	When the support of the bladder base is weakened, the bladder falls below the uterus and causes the anterior vaginal wall to bulge. The bladder also herniates into the vagina, particularly when coughing, lifting and defaecating
Cytokines (*Sigh-toe-kines*)	Small proteins which act to pass signals between cells
Cytoplasm (*Sigh-toe-pla-zim*)	A clear substance that consists of all of the contents outside of the nucleus of a membrane bound cell

Key

Primarily associated with anatomy and physiology

Primarily associated with pathophysiology

Term	Definition
Cytoskeleton (*Sigh-toe-skeleton*)	A dynamic network of fibres made of protein microfilaments and microtubules to form an internal framework of the cell, allowing movement
Cytosol (*Sigh-toe-zol*)	The aqueous component of the cytoplasm of a cell, within which various organelles and substances are suspended
Cytotoxic (*Sigh-toe-toc-sic*)	Toxic to living cells
Cytotoxic antibiotics	*See* Anti-tumour antibiotics
Cytotoxic T cells/ lymphocytes (*Lim-pho-sites*)	T lymphocytes that destroy cancer cells, cells infected by viruses or cells that are damaged
Deamination (*Dee-am-in-a-shun*)	The process by which amino acids are broken down if there is an excess of protein intake
Debridement (*Dee-bride-ment*)	Removal of dead, damaged, or infected tissue to facilitate healing
Decubitus ulcer (*De-cube-it-us ul-ser*)	A wound that occurs in the upper layers of the skin secondary to sustained, externally applied pressure that causes localised ischaemia and an inflammatory response
Deep vein thrombosis (DVT)	When a thrombus (clot) develops in a deep vein (usually lower leg); it can potentially move and occlude a blood vessel (as an embolus)
Dehydration	A condition that results from excessive loss of water from body tissues
Delayed ejaculation (*E-jack-you-lay-shun*)	A delay in orgasmic response and subsequent ejaculation despite sufficient sexual stimulation

Term	Definition
Delayed-type mediated hypersensitivity (DTH)	The activation of CD4+ T helper cells and the secretion of cytokines that promote an inflammatory reaction in people who are sensitised to an antigen, 24–72 hours after exposure
Demyelination (*Dee-my-eh-lin-a-shun*)	Loss or destruction of myelin around the axon of neurons
Dendritic cell (*Den-drit-ick*)	Antigen-presenting cells
Dendritic spine (*Den-drit-ick*)	A small membranous protrusion from a neuronal dendrite that receives input from a single axon at the synapse
Denervation (*De-ner-vay-shun*)	Loss of nerve supply
Dentine (*Den-teen*)	Hard, porous material that makes up the bulk of the tooth
Deoxyribonucleic Acid (DNA) (*Dee-ox-e-ri-bo-new-kley-ick*)	A nucleic acid molecule consisting of two polynucleotide chains in the form of a double helix that plays a central role in protein synthesis and is responsible for the transmission of hereditary characteristics
Depolarisation (*Dee-po-lar-eye-zay-shun*)	Reversal of the resting electrical potential in the neuronal cell membrane when stimulated

Key

Primarily associated with anatomy and physiology

Primarily associated with pathophysiology

Term	Definition
Depression	A neurological disorder characterised by low mood, a loss of pleasure or interest, reduced energy and feelings of guilt or low self-worth secondary to pathophysiological changes in the amygdala, hippocampus and prefrontal cortex
Dermatitis (Der-ma-tie-tis)	An inflammatory condition of the skin associated with epidermal barrier dysfunction
Dermatome (Der-ma-tome)	An area of skin normally supplied by a single spinal nerve
Dermis (Der-miss)	Layer of the skin below the epidermis
Descending (efferent) neurons (Ef-er-ent)	Neurons that carry instructions down the spinal cord from the brain to the muscles and glands of the body
Descriptive epidemiology (Ep-e-dee-me-ol-oh-gee)	Health and disease and their trends over time in specific populations
Desquamation (De-squa-may-shun)	To shed the surface keratinised cells from the stratum corneum
Detrusor (De-true-zor)	Main muscle of the bladder formed from smooth muscle fibres in spiral, longitudinal and circular bundles which empties the bladder with contraction
Detumescence (De-tomb-es-ence)	The subsiding of an erection
Diabetes insipidus (DI) (Die-ah-bee-tees in-sip-id-us)	A condition where there is insufficient secretion of or a lack of response to ADH (antidiuretic hormone), resulting in polyuria

Term	Definition
Diabetes mellitus (DM) (*Die-ah-bee-tees mel-eye-tus*)	A chronic, life-long condition of glucose metabolism in which the body responds abnormally to insulin (insulin resistance) or does not produce enough insulin to control the blood glucose level. There are two main categories of DM: • Type 1: characterised by the destruction of pancreatic beta cells and can be subdivided into two categories: type 1A (immune-mediated diabetes) and type 1B (idiopathic diabetes). This results in insulin dependence as no or very little insulin is produced. • Type 2: characterised by an inadequate amount of insulin being produced or insulin resistance.
Diabetic autonomic neuropathy (*Die-ah-bet-ick awh-toe-nom-ick nur-op-oh-thee*)	A complication associated with diabetes, it is a form of peripheral neuropathy, i.e. damage to either parasympathetic or sympathetic nerves or both
Diabetic fibrous mastopathy (*Die-ah-bet-ick fi-brus maz-top-ah-thee*)	Tough, benign masses that develop in breast tissue; a complication of type 1 diabetes mellitus
Diabetic ketoacidosis (DKA) (*Die-ah-bet-ick key-toe-ah-sid-oh-sus*)	A complication of type 1 diabetes mellitus when the body begins to break down fat for energy, producing ketones, as it is unable to use glucose because of a lack of insulin
Diaphoresis (*Die-ah-for-e-sis*)	Excessive perspiration

Key

Primarily associated with anatomy and physiology

Primarily associated with pathophysiology

Term	Definition
Diaphragm (*Die-ah-fram*)	A dome-shaped sheet of skeletal muscle that forms the floor of the thoracic cavity innervated by the phrenic nerve and used as one of the primary muscles of respiration
Diaphysis (*Die-ah-fi-sis*)	The shaft and main portion of a bone
Diarrhoea (*Die-ah-re-ah*)	The excessive passage of loose, watery stools
Diarthrosis (*Die-ar-thro-sis*)	Freely moveable joint
Diastole (*Die-ah-stol-ee*)	Relaxation of the heart muscle following a heartbeat
Diastolic dysfunction (*Die-ah-stol-ick*)	When the myocardium loses elasticity and therefore has reduced filling
Diencephalon (*Die-en-kef-a-lon*)	Part of the brain composed of the thalamus, hypothalamus, and epithalamus
Differentiation (cellular) (*Dif-er-en-see-a-shun*)	The process by which a less specialised cell becomes more specialised
Diffuse axonal injury (DAI) (*Axe-oh-nal*)	Neuronal axonal damage from a variety of mechanisms; mechanical breaking/shearage of the axonal cytoskeleton, transport disruption along the axon, inflammation of the neuronal axon, or through secondary pathophysiological changes
Diffusion (*Di-few-shun*)	The movement of ions and molecules from an area of high concentration to an area of low concentration in an attempt to achieve an isotonic balance

Term	Definition
Digestion	Breaking down food into individual nutrients both mechanically and chemically
Dilated cardiomyopathy (*Die-lay-tid kar-dee-oh-my-op-ah-thee*)	Cardiomyopathy in which the heart becomes dilated, which results in the walls of the myocardium thinning with a consequent impaired ability to pump
Diploid (*Dip-loyd*)	Two complete sets of chromosomes (46)
Direct cell-mediated response	When CD8+ cytotoxic T lymphocytes directly kill target cells expressing foreign antigens
Disability-adjusted life years	The number of years of possible life lost as a result of premature mortality and the years of productive life lost due to disability/illness
Disaccharides (*Die-sack-ah-rides*)	Carbohydrates composed of two monosaccharides
Disease	A state of disordered physiological functioning; disordered homeostasis
Dislocation	Loss of contact between the articulating surfaces of two bones at a joint
Disseminated intravascular coagulation (DIC) (*Dis-em-in-a-ted*)	Systemic activation of coagulation whereby fibrin is generated and deposited, causing microvascular thrombi in various organs that can lead to multiple organ dysfunction syndrome (MODS)

Key

Primarily associated with anatomy and physiology

Primarily associated with pathophysiology

Term	Definition
Distribution	In pharmacokinetics, distribution is the reversible movement of a drug between blood and interstitial and intracellular fluids (extravascular tissues), normally through passive diffusion
Distributive shock	A form of shock in which there is a disturbance in the distribution of circulatory volume through bypassing capillaries or pooling in capillary beds
Diverticula (*Die-ver-tic-you-la*) Plural diverticulae	Herniations (protrusions) of mucosa and submucosa through muscle layers and occur primarily in the wall of the sigmoid colon
Diverticulitis (*Die-ver-tic-you-lie-tis*)	Inflammation of the diverticula in the large intestine
DNA methylation (*Meth-ih-lay-shun*)	An epigenetic mechanism involving the addition of a methyl (CH_3) group to DNA, modifying the function and expression of genes
Dominant inheritance	When only one allele is required for the trait to be observed
Dopamine (*Doh-pa-mean*)	A neurotransmitter of the catecholamine type
Dopaminergic (*Doh-pa-min-er-jic*)	Releasing or involving dopamine
Dorsiflexion (*Dor-sea-fleck-shun*)	Movement that elevates the foot
Double-inlet ventricle	When more than half of both atria are joined to one dominant ventricle either through two separate atrioventricular (AV) valves or a common AV valve

Term	Definition
Duchenne muscular dystrophy (DMD) (*Do-shayne mus-cue-lar dis-tro-fee*)	An X-linked recessive type of muscular dystrophy caused by a mutation in the dystrophin gene that results in a lack of dystrophin, a protein, causing fibres to tear. Free calcium enters muscle cells, causing degeneration and necrosis, with skeletal muscle fibres being replaced with fat and connective tissue. The muscle increases in size with a subsequent reduction in muscle strength and function
Duct	A channel/tube leading from an exocrine gland or organ
Ductus arteriosus (*Duck-tus ar-tear-e-oh-sus*)	A blood vessel connecting the main pulmonary artery to the proximal descending aorta that permits blood from the right ventricle to bypass the fetal lungs
Ductus (vas) deferens (*Duck-tus deaf-er-ens*)	A 40-45cm (16inch) long tube that ascends out of the scrotum into the pelvic cavity, via the inguinal canal, terminating behind the bladder where it widens and joins the duct of the seminal vesicles
Duodenum (*Dew-oh-de-num*)	First part of the small intestine connecting the stomach to the jejunum
Dura Mater (*Dew-ra*)	Outermost layer of the brain and spinal cord that prevents friction against the skull, and is a lining that retains CSF within the CNS

Key

Primarily associated with anatomy and physiology

Primarily associated with pathophysiology

Term	Definition
Dynamic equilibrium (*Eck-we-lib-re-um*)	Maintenance of the body position in response to sudden movements and is perceived through rotational movement
Dysarthria (*Dis-ar-three-ah*)	Difficulty in forming words or speaking them because of weakness of muscles used in speaking or because of disruption in the neuromotor stimulus patterns required for accuracy and velocity of speech
Dysbiosis (*Dis-bi-oh-sis*)	Microbial imbalance/maladaptation in the gastrointestinal tract
Dyscalculia (*Dis-kal-cue-ley-ah*)	Difficulty with mathematics
Dyslipidaemia (*Dis-lip-id-e-me-ah*)	Distorted lipoprotein cholesterol
Dysmenorrhoea (*Dis-men-or-e-ah*)	Painful menstruation with associated abdominal cramps
Dysmetria (*Dis-me-tree-ah*)	Inability to judge distance and when to stop
Dyspareunia (*Dis-par-eh-you-knee-ah*)	Difficult or painful sexual intercourse
Dysphagia (*Dis-fay-ghee-ah*)	Difficulty in swallowing
Dysphasia (*Dys-phase-eh-ah*)	Language disorder. Inability to speak words which one has in mind or to think of correct words; or inability to understand spoken or written words. Expressive – partial or total loss of producing language in different modes (spoken, manual, or written), comprehension usually intact. Receptive – people have difficulty understanding written and spoken language

Term	Definition
Dysphonia (*Dis-fo-knee-ah*)	Difficulty in speaking due to a physical impairment of the mouth, tongue, throat, or vocal cords
Dysplasia (*Dis-play-zee-ah*)	A condition in which the cells of a particular tissue vary in size and shape, mitosis is increased, and large cell nuclei are seen
Dyspnoea (*Dis-knee-ah*)	Difficulty in breathing
Dysuria (*Dis-you-ree-ah*)	Painful or difficult urination
Eburnation (*Eh-bur-nay-shun* or *E-bur-nay-shun*)	Conversion of bone or cartilage, through thinning or loss, into a hard, dense mass with a polished, ivory-like finish
Ecchymotic (*Eck-e-mo-tic*)	Discolouration (black/blue) of tissue due to extravasation of blood, e.g. bruising
Eccrine (merocrine) gland (*Eh-krin (mer-oh-krin)*)	Most common sweat gland in the skin with ducts that open onto the surface of the skin and produce a clear, watery sweat
Eclampsia (*E-klamp-see-ah*)	A condition whereby a pregnant woman develops neurological disturbances and seizures secondary to hypertension (has pre-eclampsia)
Ectasia (*Eck-tay-see-ah* or *Eck-tay-sha*)	Dilation or distention of tubular structures, including blood vessels
Ectopic (*Eck-top-ick*)	In an abnormal place or position

Key

Primarily associated with anatomy and physiology

Primarily associated with pathophysiology

Term	Definition
Ectopic pregnancy	Pregnancy in which the fetus develops outside the uterus, usually within a Fallopian tube
Eczema (*Eck-zee-ma or eck-se-ma*)	*See* Dermatitis
Ejaculation (*E-jack-you-lay-shun*)	The action of expelling semen from the body
Ejaculatory duct (*E-jack-you-lay-tor-e*)	A short 2 cm (1 inch) duct that passes through the prostate gland and merges with the urethra
Ejaculatory dysfunction	Sexual dysfunction of ejaculation in men that includes premature ejaculation, delayed ejaculation and retrograde ejaculation
Ejection fraction	The volume, or percentage, of blood pumped (or ejected) out of the ventricles with each contraction
Elastin (*E-las-tin*)	An elastic, fibrous glycoprotein in connective tissue
Electrolyte (*E-lec-tro-light*)	A substance that dissociates into ions when dissolved in a solution and attains the ability to conduct electricity
Element	A pure chemical substance consisting of a single type of atom
Elimination (*E-lim-in-a-shun*)	The act of removing waste products from the body
Embolism (*Em-bow-liz-im*) Plural emboli	When an embolus occludes a blood vessel
Embolus (*Em-bow-lus*)	A blood clot, air bubble, segment of fatty deposit, or other substance carried in the bloodstream that lodges in and occludes a vessel

Term	Definition
Embryo (*Em-bree-oh*)	The collection of cells that has developed from the fertilised egg before all the major organs have developed fully and differentiated fully. The embryo becomes a fetus eight weeks after fertilisation
Emesis (*Em-ih-sis*)	The forceful expulsion of chyme (stomach and/or intestinal contents) through the mouth (act of vomiting)
Emphysema (*Em-phe-see-ma*)	An obstructive airway disease characterised by destructive changes of the alveolar walls and irreversible enlargement of the alveolar sacs with loss of surface area for gaseous exchange
Empyema (*Em-pie-e-ma*)	Accumulation of pus in a body cavity
Enamel (*E-nah-mel*)	Hard, bone like structure that protects the tooth
Encephalitis (*En-kef-ah-lie-tis*)	Inflammation of the brain parenchyma
Endarterectomy (*En-dar-ter-eck-toe-me*)	An endovascular procedure to remove atheromatous plaques in the lining of an artery
Endemic (*En-dem-ick*)	When a condition is generally present in a group or area
Endocardium (*En-doh-kar-de-um*)	Innermost layer of the heart muscle forming the lining of the heart and heart valves
Endocrine glands (*En-do-cryne*)	Ductless glands that release hormones directly into the blood stream

Key

Primarily associated with anatomy and physiology

Primarily associated with pathophysiology

Term	Definition
Endocytosis (*En-doh-sigh-toe-sis*)	Energy-using process by which cells absorb molecules (such as proteins) by engulfing them by means of a coated vacuole or vesicle
Endolymph (*En-doh-limph*)	Fluid within the cochlear duct (scala media)
Endometriosis (*En-doh-me-tree-oh-sis*)	A condition in which functional endometrial tissue, normally within the uterine cavity, is found in sites outside the uterus, usually the ovaries, fallopian tubes, other organs of the reproductive system, uterosacral ligaments, intestines and pelvic organs
Endometrium (*En-doh-me-tree-um*)	The mucous membrane lining the uterus that thickens during the menstrual cycle for possible implantation of an embryo
Endoplasmic reticulum (*En-doh-plaz-mick*)	A cell-wide network of interconnected, flattened, membrane-enclosed sacs spread throughout a cell which provide a surface on which lipids and proteins can be formed and transported around the cell. There are two types; smooth and rough
Endospore (*En-doh-spore*)	Highly resistant structures that can remain dormant for many years and are resistant to desiccation, toxic chemicals and UV irradiation. When conditions become favourable, they become active and germinate
Endosteum (*En-doz-tee-um*)	Single layer of bone producing cells lining the inner surfaces of the cavities within bone
Endothelial cells (*En-doh-thee-lee-al*)	Cells that line the interior surface of blood and lymphatic vessels

Term	Definition
Endothelins (*En-doh-thee-lins*)	Peptides which are major regulators of vascular tone and blood pressure
Endothelium (*En-doh-thee-lee-um*)	The tissue formed by a single layer of cells, lining various organs and body cavities
Endotoxin (*En-doh-tocks-in*)	Toxic substance bound to the wall of gram-negative bacteria
Engorgement (*En-gorge-ment*)	When an organ or tissue is filled with blood or fluid to the point of congestion/capacity
Enteral (*En-ter-al*)	Involving or passing through the gastrointestinal tract (e.g. through oral ingestion or tube feeding)
Enterocele (*En-ter-oh-seal*)	When a portion of the small bowel descends into the space between the posterior surface of the vagina and the anterior surface of the rectum
Enteroreceptors (*En-ter-oh-re-cep-tors*)	Sensory receptors in the internal environment
Enterotoxins (*En-ter-oh-tocks-ins*)	Specific exotoxins that affect the gastrointestinal tract
Enzyme (*En-zyme*)	Biological catalyst
Eosinophils (*Ee-o-sin-o-fils*)	Granulocytes that function in allergic responses and in resisting some infections by engulfing antigen-antibody complexes, allergens and inflammatory chemicals. They also weaken or kill parasites by secreting chemical agents

Key

Primarily associated with anatomy and physiology

Primarily associated with pathophysiology

Term	Definition
Ependymal cells (*Eh-pen-die-mal*)	Neuroglia that form the epithelial lining of the ventricles of the brain which create and secrete CSF and circulate it by cilia activity
Epidemic (*Epp-eh-dem-ick*)	Widespread distribution of a condition in a specific area at a specific time
Epidemiology (*Ep-e-dee-me-ol-oh-gee*)	The scientific study of health and disease in populations to understand the range of factors which influence the distribution of disease through the population and how it spreads between populations
Epidermis (*Epp-e-der-mis*)	The thin, outermost layer of the skin
Epidermoid cysts (*Epp-e-der-moid*)	Dome-shaped lesions of the pilosebaceous follicle largely formed as a result of infection; they are benign encapsulated, subepidermal nodules filled with keratin
Epidermolysis bullosa acquisita (EBA) (*Epp-e-der-mo-lie-sis bull-oh-sa ah-quee-sit-ah*)	A heterogeneous organ-specific autoimmune disease that occurs when autoantibodies to type VII collagen are induced, causing mucocutaneous blisters
Epididymis (*Epp-e-did-ih-mus*)	A six-metre coiled and convoluted tube on the posterior border of the testis consisting of 12 ducts which carry, mature, store and release sperm
Epididymitis (*Epp-e-did-ih-my-tis*)	Infection or inflammation of the epididymis
Epididymo-orchitis (*Epp-e-did-ih-mo or-ki-tis*)	Infection or inflammation of the epididymis and the testes
Epigenetic therapy (*Epp-e-gen-et-ick*)	The use of drugs that inhibit DNA methylation and histone deacetylation, thereby reversing epigenetic modifications

Term	Definition
Epigenetics (*Epp-e-gen-et-icks*)	The study of changes caused by modification of gene expression rather than alteration of the genetic code itself
Epiglottis (*Epp-e-glot-is*)	A thin, cartilaginous flap that covers the glottis during swallowing, preventing swallowed substances entering the larynx
Epilepsy (*Eh-pil-ep-see*)	A distinct, chronic seizure disorder characterised by an imbalance between excitatory and inhibitory neurotransmitter activity in cerebral neuronal ions. A tendency toward recurrent seizures unprovoked by any systemic or acute neurologic insults
Epileptogenesis (*Eh-pee-lep-toe-jen-ih-sis*)	Sequence of events that converts a normal neuronal network into a hyperexcitable network that leads to the development of spontaneous recurrent seizures
Epiphyses (*Eh-pif-ih-seas*)	The proximal and distal ends of a bone
Epithalamus (*Epp-e-thal-a-mus*)	Relay centre composed primarily of the pineal gland and the habenula
Epithelial cells (*Epp-e-thee-lee-al*)	Cells of the epithelium
Epithelial tissue	Tissue that covers the body and lines cavities, organs, and glands
Epithelium (*Epp-e-thee-lee-um*)	A membranous cellular tissue that covers the surface or lines a tube or cavity of body structure

Key

Primarily associated with anatomy and physiology

Primarily associated with pathophysiology

Term	Definition
Equilibrium (*Eh-qui-lib-re-um*)	The sense that helps maintain balance and awareness of orientation in space (proprioception)
Erectile dysfunction (ED) (*E-rec-tile dis-funk-shun*)	A complex condition that occurs secondary to neural, vascular and/or hormonal dysfunction that impairs penile erection
Erythrocytes (*E-rith-ro-sites*)	Red blood cells – the most abundant blood cell, formed in the red bone marrow and containing the pigment haemoglobin which transports oxygen and carbon dioxide to and from the cells of the body. Each erythrocyte has approximately 280 million haemoglobin molecules, and so can carry four times that amount of oxygen
Erythrocytosis (*E-rith-ro-sigh-toe-sis*)	An increase in the number of circulating erythrocytes
Erythropoiesis (*E-rith-ro-po-e-sus*)	Formation of new erythrocytes
Erythropoietin (EPO) (*E-rith-ro-po-e-tin*)	A hormone produced by the kidneys that stimulates the red bone marrow to produce more erythrocytes
Essential hypertension	*See* Primary hypertension
Eukaryotes (*You-car-e-oh-cites*)	These include both animal and vegetable, and single and multiple-celled organisms with more complex cells that have a nuclear membrane surrounding the characteristic defining chromosomes
Euploidy (*You-ploy-dee*)	When a cell has any number of complete chromosome sets (an exact multiple of the haploid number)

Term	Definition
Eustachian (auditory) tube (*You-stay-shun*)	Tube that connects the nasopharynx and tympanic cavity and opens to allow air to move in to equalise air pressure on either side of the tympanic membrane
Evaluative epidemiology	Evaluates preventative interventions, estimates risk of specific diseases for people exposed to hazards
Evaporation (*E-vap-or-ray-shun*)	The conversion of a liquid to vapour resulting in a loss of heat energy
Eversion (*E-ver-shun*)	Turning the sole of the foot outwards, inner side of foot on the ground
Excitotoxicity (*Eck-sigh-toe-tocks-is-it-e*)	The pathophysiological process whereby neurons are damaged and killed by overactivation of receptors for excitatory glutamate (neurotransmitter): intracellular organelles are damaged, leading to death of the neuron
Excretion (*Ex-cree-shun*)	A process of eliminating metabolic waste from an organism
Exocrine glands (*Ex-oh-crine*)	Glands that release hormones through ducts to the surface of an organ or into a cavity
Exocytosis (*Ex-oh-sigh-toe-sis*)	The release of cellular substances by fusing the vesicular membrane with the plasma membrane and subsequently expelling the substances out of the cell
Extension	Movement that increases the angle/distance between two bones or parts of body

Key

Primarily associated with anatomy and physiology

Primarily associated with pathophysiology

Term	Definition
External respiration	The diffusion of gases between the alveoli and the pulmonary capillaries across the respiratory membrane
Exteroreceptors (*Ex-ter-oh-re-sep-tors*)	Sensory receptors in the external environment located in the skin
Extracellular fluid (ECF) (*Ex-tra-sell-u-lar*)	Fluid outside of cells made up of plasma (the fluid component of blood) and interstitial/intercellular fluid (fluid between cells)
Extracellular matrix (*Ex-tra-sell-u-lar may-tricks*)	Collection of substances outside of cells that provide structural and biochemical support to the surrounding cells, enabling them to 'stick' together. These cells have a crucial role to play in wound healing as they produce collagen
Extracorporeal life support (ECLS) (*Ex-tra-kor-pour-e-al*)	The use of equipment external to the body to carry out the functions of a non-functioning organ
Extradural (epidural) haematoma (*Ex-tra-due-ral (Epp-e-due-ral) (Hay-ma-toe-ma or Heem-ma-toe-ma*)	A collection of blood between the skull and the dura mater when a force has resulted in periosteal dura mater-bone cleavage
Extraembryonic (*Ex-tra-em-bree-on-ick*)	Referring to outside of the embryo
Extrinsic (*Ex-trin-sick*)	Originating outside or/external to
Fabry disease (*Pha-bri*)	Deficiency of an enzyme alpha-galactosidase A
Facioscapulohumeral muscular dystrophy (FSHD) (*Phash-e-oh-sca-pew-low-hue-mer-al*)	An autosomal dominant inherited form of muscular dystrophy in which muscles of the limbs, shoulders and face weaken

Term	Definition
Facultative aerobes (*Fa-kul-tay-tive aer-robes*)	Microorganisms that can grow if oxygen is available or not
Faecalith (*Fee-kal-ith*)	Hard piece of stool/faeces
Failure to thrive	Insufficient weight gain or inappropriate weight loss
Falciform ligament (*Fal-see-form*)	Ligament dividing the liver into the left and right lobes
Fallopian tube (*Fal-oh-pea-an*)	A pair of tubes along which the ovum travels from the ovaries to the uterus
Farber disease	An inherited disorder of lipid metabolism associated with the deficiency of the enzyme ceramidase and accumulation of ceramide in the lysosome
Fascia (*Fash-e-ah*)	A band or sheet of subcutaneous tissue that anchors, encloses, and separates muscles and other internal organs
Fat	A macronutrient composed of glycerol and fatty acid combinations
Fauces (*Faw-sees*)	The opening from the oral cavity into the oropharynx
Femur (*Fee-mur*)	The longest and strongest bone in the body located in the upper leg
Fertilisation	The fusion of two gametes (sex cells)
Fetus (*Fee-tus*)	A human embryo is called a fetus from the end of the second month of pregnancy until birth. At this stage, differentiation becomes more distinct and vital organs develop further and become active

Key

Primarily associated with anatomy and physiology

Primarily associated with pathophysiology

Term	Definition
Fibre (*Fi-bur*)	A non-starch polysaccharide (or cellulose) composed of oligosaccharides and polysaccharides
Fibrin (*Fi-brin*)	An insoluble protein formed from fibrinogen during blood clotting that forms a fibrous web in haemostasis
Fibrinogen (*Fi-brin-oh-jen*)	A glycoprotein involved in blood clotting
Fibrinolytic (*Fi-brin-oh-lit-ick*)	Processes or substance that result in the disintegration or dissolution of fibrin, usually through enzymatic action
Fibrinopurulent (*Fi-brin-oh-purr-you-lent*)	Pus or exudate that contain a relatively large amount of fibrin
Fibroadenomas (*Fi-bro-ad-en-oh-mas*)	Benign breast tumours composed of glandular and stromal (connective) tissue
Fibroatheroma (*Fi-bro-ath-er-oma*)	A lipid-rich necrotic core encapsulated by collagen rich fibrous tissue. An advanced lesion of coronary atherosclerosis
Fibroblasts (*Fi-bro-blasts*)	Cells that synthesise the extracellular matrix and collagen
Fibrocystic changes (*Fi-bro-sis-tick*)	Non-malignant changes in the breasts that include breast pain, cysts, and lumpiness
Fibroids (*Fi-broids*)	*See* Leiomyomas
Fibroma (*Fi-bro-ma*)	A benign fibrous tumour of connective tissue

Term	Definition
Fibromyalgia (*Fi-bro-my-al-gee-ah*)	A chronic syndrome affecting the musculoskeletal system that is characterised by widespread pain, increased sensitivity to touch, fatigue, non-restorative sleep, anxiety and depression
Fibrosis (*Fi-bro-sis*)	Thickening and scarring of connective tissue, usually as a result of injury
Fibrous joint (*Fi-brus*)	Type of joint where two bones are attached by fibrous connective tissue
Fibula (*Fib-you-la*)	Bone running parallel to the tibia on the outside of the lower leg
Filtration	The movement of water, ions, and molecules from an area of higher pressure to an area of lower pressure, usually across a semipermeable membrane, due to the hydrostatic pressure of the fluid
First pass metabolism	The metabolism of a proportion of a drug administered before it reaches the systemic circulation (usually due to passage through the liver)
Fissure (*Fish-ure*)	A groove or cleft (normal or abnormal) on the surface of an organ or bony structure
Flaccid paralysis (*Fla-sid*)	Weakness and loss of muscle tone secondary to lower motor neuron dysfunction
Flexion (*Fleck-shun*)	Movement that decreases the angle of a joint
Flora (*Flor-ah*)	The microorganisms (bacteria or fungi) living in or on the body

Key

Primarily associated with anatomy and physiology

Primarily associated with pathophysiology

Term	Definition
Follicle (*Fol-ick-al*)	A secretory cavity, sac, or gland
Follicle stimulating hormone (FSH)	A hormone that activates Sertoli cells in men, and stimulates the growth of ovarian follicles in women
Follicular cells (*Fol-ick-you-lar*)	These are also known as thyroid epithelial cells and are located in the thyroid gland where they produce and secrete thyroxine (T_4) and triiodothyronine (T_3)
Foramen magnum (*Four-a-men mag-numb*)	Opening in the base of the skull through which the spinal cord passes
Foramen magnum decompression	Removal of suboccipital bone to increase space and allow CSF to flow
Foramen of Monro	Connection between the third ventricle and the lateral ventricles
Foramen ovale (*Four-a-men oh-val-eh*)	An opening in the septum between the two atria of the heart that is normally patent only in the fetus
Forebrain	Largest section of the brain consisting of the diencephalon and the cerebrum
Foreskin (prepuce) (*pre-pews*)	The skin over the penile glans
Fovea centralis (*Fov-e-ah sen-tra-lis*)	Located near the optic disc, this is an area of high density cones and is responsible for detailed images
Fracture	Break or disruption in the continuity of a bone
Fragility fracture	A fracture of a bone from a fall or bump that would not ordinarily have caused a bone to break
Free nerve endings	General sensory receptors that respond to temperature changes of heat and cold, as well as pain

Term	Definition
Frenulum (*Fren-you-lum*)	Fold of tissue where the foreskin attaches to the penile glans
Fucosidosis (*Phew-co-sid-oh-sis*)	A lysosomal storage disease
Fundus (*Fun-dus*)	Part of a hollow organ (such as the uterus or the gallbladder) that is furthest from the opening. Also refers to the upper part of the stomach
Fungi (*Fun-gee*)	Any of a wide variety of single or multi-cell organisms that reproduce by spores, including the mushrooms, moulds, yeasts and mildews
Galactokinase deficiency (*Ga-lack-toe-kin-aze*)	A genetic metabolic disorder characterised by an accumulation of galactose and galactitol as a result of decreased conversion of galactose to galactose-1-phosphate by galactokinase
Galactorrhoea (*Ga-lack-toe-ree-ah*)	Spontaneous milk secretion
Galactosaemia (*Ga-lact-toe-see-me-ah*)	An inherited disorder of galactose metabolism that primarily occurs in newborn children
Gallbladder	Small sac located at the underside of the liver that stores and concentrates bile
Gamete (*Ga-meet*)	A mature reproductive cell having a single set of chromosomes
Gamma-Aminobutyric Acid (GABA) (*Ga-ma a-mean-oh-bew-tir-ick*)	An inhibitory neurotransmitter that blocks the transmission of nerve impulses in the central nervous system

Key

Primarily associated with anatomy and physiology

Primarily associated with pathophysiology

Term	Definition
Ganglion (*Gang-ley-on*)	A cluster of neurons or neuronal cell bodies in the peripheral nervous system
Gangliosidoses (*Gang-ley-oh-sid-oh-sis*)	Group of disorders of accumulation of lipids known as gangliosides
Gangrene (*Gang-reen*)	Tissue death secondary to inadequate blood supply
Gaseous exchange	The process that occurs in alveoli where oxygen is extracted from inhaled air into the bloodstream and carbon dioxide is extracted from the blood for elimination through exhalation
Gastritis (*Gas-try-tis*)	Inflammation of the gastric mucosa
Gastrointestinal tract (GIT) (*Gas-tro-in-tes-tin-al*)	A hollow tube which runs from the mouth to the anus with the purpose of moving nutrients from the external environment into the internal environment and eliminating ingested waste products
Gastro-oesophageal reflux disease (GORD/GERD) (*Gas-tro-oh-sof-ih-gee-al*)	Persistent reflux of stomach contents, i.e. acid, pepsin and bile salts, into the oesophagus causing oesophagitis
Gaucher disease (*Gau-sher*)	A genetic disorder of metabolism where glucocerebroside (a lipid) cannot be adequately broken down
Gender identity	The sense of being male or female
Gender role	How people behave as men or women (as society perceives them)
Gene expression	The process by which specific genes are activated to produce a required protein, i.e. the functional gene product

Term	Definition
Gene therapy	*Using genes* to treat or prevent disease by inserting gene into patient's cells. *Or* the use of drugs that suppress overactive oncogenes to activate tumour suppressor genes
General senses	The sensations of pain, temperature, light touch and pressure
Genes *(Jeans)*	Section of DNA which codes for a specific polypeptide chain
Genetics *(Jen-eh-ticks)*	Refers to specific individual genes and how they are inherited
Genomics *(Jen-om-icks)*	Refers to the complete genetic makeup of an individual and how it interacts with environmental and lifestyle factors
Genotype *(Jen-oh-type)*	The overall structure of an individual's genetic makeup
Germline mosaicism *(Mow-zay-ick-ism)*	When some germline cells have a normal chromosomal make-up while others carry a chromosome change
Gestation *(Jes-tay-shun)*	The process or period of development from conception to birth
Gestational hypertension *(Jes-tay-shon-al hi-per-ten-shun)*	Hypertension that occurs after 20 weeks of gestation but there are no other signs of pre-eclampsia and disappears within three months of delivery
Gestational trophoblastic disease *(Jes-tay-shon-al tro-fo-blas-tick)*	A group of disorders in which tumours grow in the uterus during pregnancy

Key

Primarily associated with anatomy and physiology

Primarily associated with pathophysiology

Term	Definition
Ghon complex (*Gone*)	The collective term for the primary lung lesion and lymph node granulomas in tuberculosis
Ghon focus	A granulomatous lesion containing tubercle bacilli, modified macrophages and other immune cells
Ghrelin (*Gre-lyn*)	The 'hunger hormone' produced by cells in the stomach which enhances the sensation of feeling hungry before an expected meal
Gilbert's syndrome	A genetic disorder of bilirubin metabolism
Glans	The rounded head of a penis
Gleason score (*Glee-sun*)	The sum of two scales scored 1 to 5 that designates the degree of differentiation of the tumour of the prostate gland predominant cell lines
Gliadin (*Gly-a-din*)	A protein that is a component of gluten
Gliosis (*Gly-oh-sis*)	A fibrous proliferation of glial cells in injured areas of the CNS leading to scar tissue formation
Global aphasia (*A-phase-e-ah*)	When a person will produce few recognisable words and understand little or no spoken language. They can also neither read nor write
Globulins (*Glob-you-lins*)	Proteins essential for immunity with some functioning as antibodies against infection while others transport some hormones and minerals
Glomerular filtration rate (GFR) (*Glom-er-you-lar*)	The rate at which the filtrate is formed in the Bowman's capsule of the kidneys, measured in millilitres per minute

Term	Definition
Glomerulonephritis (*Glom-er-you-low-nef-rye-tis*)	Inflammation of the renal glomeruli
Glomerulosclerosis (*Glom-er-you-low-scler-oh-sis*)	Formation of scar tissue in glomeruli
Glomerulus (*Glom-er-you-lus*)	Tiny tufts of capillaries which carry blood within the kidneys
Glucagon (*Glue-ka-gon*)	A peptide hormone that raises blood glucose level when it falls too low by stimulating conversion of glycogen in the liver into glucose
Glucocorticoids (*Glue-ko-kor-ti-koyds*)	Any of a group of anti-inflammatory corticosteroids involved in the metabolism of carbohydrates, proteins, and fats
Gluconeogenesis (*Glue-ko-knee-oh-gen-ih-sis*)	Production of glucose from lactate, amino acids and the glycerol component of fat
Glucosuria (*Glue-kose-you-ree-a*)	*See* Glycosuria
Glutamate (*Glue-ta-mate*)	An excitatory neurotransmitter
Glycerol (*Glih-ser-ol*)	A three carbon molecule produced by hydrolysis of fats
Glycogen (*Gly-ko-gen*)	Carbohydrate store in the body

Key

Primarily associated with anatomy and physiology

Primarily associated with pathophysiology

Term	Definition
Glycogen storage disease type II	An autosomal recessive metabolic disorder whereby there is a deficiency in an enzyme (acid alpha-glucosidase (acid maltase)) needed to break down glycogen, resulting in an accumulation of glycogen in lysosomes
Glycogenesis (*Gly-ko-gen-ih-sis*)	The conversion of glucose to glycogen for storage in the liver
Glycogenolysis (*Gly-ko-gen-ol-ih-sis*)	The process by which glycogen is broken down into glucose to provide an immediate energy source
Glycolipid (*Gly-ko-lip-id*)	A molecule consisting of a carbohydrate plus a lipid
Glycolysis (*Gly-kol-ih-sis*)	Breakdown of glucose by enzymes, releasing energy and pyruvate
Glycoprotein (*Gly-ko-pro-teen*)	A molecule consisting of a carbohydrate plus a protein. Proteins which have oligosaccharide chains
Glycosuria (*Gly-kose-you-ree-ah*)	Glucose in the urine
Goblet cells	Cells that produce mucus, found in the respiratory and gastrointestinal tracts
Golgi body (*Gol-guy*)	A cell organelle composed of stacks of flattened sacs of membrane which receives proteins and lipids from the ER and packages them into secretory vesicles. These are stored and moved to the plasma membrane when needed
Golgi tendon organs	General sensory receptors that detect tension as part of proprioception
Gomphosis (*Gom-fo-sis*)	Type of fibrous joint formed with collagenous connective tissue (those between the teeth and the mandible and maxillae)

Term	Definition
Gonadal dysgenesis (*Go-na-dal dis-gen-ih-sis*)	Loss of germ cells; congenital developmental disorder of the reproductive system in the male or female
Gonadotropin-releasing hormone (GnRH) (*Go-nad-oh-tro-fin*)	A hormone secreted by the hypothalamus that triggers the anterior pituitary to release gonadotropins
Gonocytes (*Go-no-sites*)	Germ cell responsible for spermatogenesis and oogenesis
Gonorrhoea (*Gon-or-eh-ah*)	A sexually transmitted infection caused by *Neisseria gonorrhoeae*, a gram-negative diplococcus bacterium that is spread by direct contact with the mucosa of an infected individual
Gout	A syndrome that results in hyperuricaemia caused by either increased uric acid production or decreased uric acid excretion by the kidneys leading to uric acid deposition in joints
Granular cell tumour (*Gran-you-lar*)	A tumour (usually benign) that probably originates from Schwann cells of the peripheral nervous system
Granulation (*Gran-you-lay-shun*)	The formation of new connective tissue
Granulocytes (*Gran-you-low-sites*)	Leucocytes that have visible granules, which are the organelles, in the cytoplasm

Key

Primarily associated with anatomy and physiology

Primarily associated with pathophysiology

Term	Definition
Granuloma (*Gran-you-low-ma*)	A mass of granulation tissue that occurs in response to infection, inflammation, or the presence of a foreign body
Granulomatous (*Gran-you-low-ma-tus*)	Of, relating to, or characterised by granuloma
Granulomatous hypersensitivity	A chronic type IV reaction where macrophages are activated in response to microbial antigens
Granulysin (*Gran-you-lie-sin*)	A cytokine which is identified as the key mediator of keratinocyte destruction through apoptosis
Graves' disease	An autoimmune condition in which the body's immune system is attacking its own tissues which stimulates growth of the thyroid gland and increased thyroid hormone secretion
Grey matter	Grouping of nerve cell bodies
Guillain-Barré syndrome (GBS) (*Ghee-yhan bar-ay*)	An acute inflammatory demyelinating polyneuropathy or an acute motor axonal neuropathy. Rapid-onset muscle weakness is caused by immune system damage of the peripheral nervous system
Gumma (*Gum-ma*)	A soft, necrotic, fibrous granuloma resulting from the tertiary stage of syphilis
Gustation (*Gus-tay-shun*)	Sensation of taste
Gyri (*Jai-re*)	Folds in the white matter of the cerebral cortex in between sulci
Habenula (*Ha-ben-you-la*)	Relay from the limbic system, and deals with sleep, stress, pain, and reinforcement processing

Term	Definition
Haematemesis (*Heem-a-tem-a-sis*)	Vomiting of blood
Haematocrit (*Heem-a-toe-crit*)	The ratio of the volume of erythrocytes to the total volume of blood
Haematogenous spread (*Heem-a-togg-en-us*)	Spread via bloodstream
Haematoma (*Heem-a-toe-ma*)	A large area of accumulated blood from a local haemorrhage
Haematopoietic (*Heem-a-toe-po-et-ick*)	Pertaining to the formation of blood or blood cells
Haematuria (*Heem-a-ture-e-ah*)	The presence of blood in urine
Haemochromatosis (*Heem-oh-chrome-ah-toe-sis*)	A genetic disorder whereby there is excess iron absorption
Haemoglobin (*Heem-oh-glow-bin*)	A protein composed of globin and haem and containing four globin chains and four haem units enabling each haemoglobin molecule to carry four oxygen molecules
Haemoglobinopathies (*Heem-oh-glow-bin-op-a-thees*)	Conditions in which there is an abnormality in structure of (one) of the globin chains of the haemoglobin molecule
Haemoglobinuria (*Heem-oh-glow-bin-you-ree-ah*)	Presence of free haemoglobin in the urine

Key

Primarily associated with anatomy and physiology

Primarily associated with pathophysiology

Term	Definition
Haemolytic anaemia (*Heem-oh-lit-ick a-knee-me-ah*)	Type of anaemia whereby erythrocytes are prematurely destroyed and eliminated
Haemophilia (*Heem-oh-fil-e-ah*)	An X-linked condition where a deficiency of clotting factors leads to an impaired ability of blood to clot
Haemopoiesis (*Heem-oh-po-e-sis*)	Production of blood cells
Haemoptysis (*Heem-op-tis-is*)	Coughing up of blood or bloody secretions
Haemorrhagic stroke (*Hae-mor-ah-jick*)	A stroke caused by the rupture of a blood vessel in the brain
Haemostasis (*Heem-oh-stay-sis*)	The process by which bleeding is stopped
Haemostasis (wound healing)	The first stage of healing, referring to the stopping of haemorrhage at the site of injury by contraction of the smooth muscle in the arterial and arteriole walls, significantly reducing the blood flow
Haemothorax (*Heem-oh-tho-racks*)	The presence of blood in the pleural cavity
Hair receptors	General sensory receptors that interpret touch by movement of hair (root hair plexus)
Half-life	The time required for any specified property, e.g. the concentration of a hormone or drug in the body, to decrease by half
Hamartoma (*Ha-mar-toe-ma*)	A benign uncommon tumour of varying amounts of glandular, adipose and fibrous tissue
Haploid (*Hap-loyd*)	One complete set of chromosomes present in gametes

Term	Definition
Hapten (*Hap-ten*)	An incomplete soluble antigen which, when combined with a larger carrier protein, is recognised as an antigen
Haustrations (*Haw-stray-shuns*)	Small segmented pouches of the colon that give it a segmented appearance and maximise surface area for absorption of water and minerals
Haustrum (*Haw-strum (haw-stra)*) Plural haustra	A structure resembling a recess or sac formation
Haversian canals (*Ha-ver-see-an*)	Minute tubes which form a network in bone and contain blood vessels
Health improvement	Interventions to improve the health and well-being of individuals or communities through facilitating the adoption of healthy lifestyle choices and tackling factors that influence health in society (poverty, social housing, education)
Health promotion	The facilitation of people to take positive, autonomous control of their health through a diverse set of approaches that improve health-related quality of life through the prevention of ill-health
Health protection	The area of public health practice concerned with actions to reduce exposure to factors which can impact on development of ill-health
Health services epidemiology	Describes and analyses work of health services

Key

Primarily associated with anatomy and physiology

Primarily associated with pathophysiology

Term	Definition
Hearing	The ability to interpret sound
Heart failure	Failure of the heart to effectively pump blood around the body, so that its ability to respond to increased demands for cardiac output is impaired
Heart rate	The number of heartbeats in one minute
Helix (*He-licks*)	Upper rim of the auricle
Helminths (*Hell-minths*)	Multi-cellular parasitic worms
Hemianopia (*Hem-e-ah-no-pee-ah*)	Blindness in one half of the visual field
Hemiparesis (*Hem-e-par-e-sis*)	Weakness down one side of the body
Hepatic artery (*Hep-at-ick*)	Branch of the coeliac artery that delivers a rich supply of oxygenated blood to the liver
Hepatic encephalopathy (*Hep-at-ick en-cef-a-lop-a-thee*)	The totality of central nervous system (CNS) manifestations of liver failure, characterised by a variety of neural disturbances
Hepatic vein	Vein carrying blood from the liver to the vena cava
Hepatitis (*Hep-a-tie-tis*)	Inflammation of the liver
Hepatocytes (*Hep-a-toe-sites*)	Functional cells of the liver
Hepatomegaly (*Hep-a-toe-meg-a-lee*)	Abnormal enlargement of the liver
Hepatopancreatic ampulla (*Hep-a-toe-pan-kree-a-tic am-pule-ah*)	Junction of the pancreatic and bile ducts as they open into the duodenum

Term	Definition
Heterogeneous (genetic) (*Het-er-oj-en-us*)	When there are mutations at two or more genetic loci that yield the same or similar phenotypes
Heteroplasmy (*Het-er-oh-plaz-me*)	When a cell has some mitochondria that have a mutation in the mitochondrial DNA and some that do not
Heterozygote screening (*Het-er-oh-zi-goat*)	Genetic testing of a population or subpopulation to identify heterozygous carriers of a disease-causing allele who are healthy but have the potential to produce children with the disease
Heterozygous (*Het-er-oh-zi-guz*)	Refers to a pair of genes where one is dominant and one is recessive
Hiatal hernia (*High-a-tal her-knee-ah*)	A diaphragmatic protrusion (herniation) of the stomach (upper part) through the diaphragm into the thorax
Hiatus hernia (*High-a-tus her-knee-ah*)	*See* Hiatal hernia
High density lipoproteins (HDLs) (*Lie-po-pro-teens*)	Type of lipoprotein that mops up cholesterol in the blood transporting it to the liver for elimination in bile
High glycaemic index carbohydrates (*Gly-see-mick*)	The index represents the relative ability of a carbohydrate food to increase the level of glucose in the blood. Foods that score highly should be avoided

Key

Primarily associated with anatomy and physiology

Primarily associated with pathophysiology

Term	Definition
Hilum (*Hill-um or High-lum*)	The point where structures such as blood vessels and nerves enter an organ
Hip bone	Unit bone of the pelvic girdle made up of the ilium, ischium and pubis bones
Hippocampus (*Hip-oh-kam-pus*)	Part of the limbic system primarily associated with formation of memory, and organising sensory and cognitive experiences for storage
Hirsutism (*Her-zoo-tis-im*)	Unwanted, male-pattern hair growth in women
Histamine (*Hiss-ta-mean*)	An inflammatory agent released by cells in response to injury/allergy/inflammation that causes dilation of capillaries and contraction of smooth muscle
Histone modification (*Hiss-tone*)	Epigenetic mechanism: post-translational modifications (modification of proteins following protein biosynthesis) that regulate gene expression
Histotoxic hypoxia (*Hiss-toe-tox-ick*)	When cells are unable to use the oxygen reaching them
Homeostasis (*Home-e-oh-stay-sis*)	Regulation of the internal environment in order that a level of consistency is maintained necessary for the cells and organs of the body to operate optimally
Homocystinuria (*Home-oh-sis-tin-your-e-ah*)	A disorder of methionine metabolism, leading to accumulation of homocysteine (an amino acid created during the metabolism of methionine and cysteine) and its metabolites in blood and urine
Homologous (*Ho-mol-oh-gus*)	Pair of autosomes, one from each parent, similar in length, gene position, and centromere location

Term	Definition
Homozygous (*Home-oh-zigh-gus*)	Having identical pairs of genes for any given pair of hereditary characteristics
Hormone antagonist (*An-tag-on-ist*)	Substances that act upon hormone receptors of cells to inhibit the endocrine function
Hormones	Chemical messengers secreted directly into the blood stream and carried around the body in the blood to attach to their specific receptor and influence the activity of the specific target cells, tissues, organs and systems of the body
Human chorionic gonadotrophin (hCG) (*Kor-e-on-ick go-nad-oh-tro-fin*)	A placental hormone that maintains the corpus luteum during pregnancy
Human Immunodeficiency Virus (HIV)	A virus that destroys the $CD4^+$ cells of the immune system and suppresses the immune response. It can cause Acquired Immunodeficiency Syndrome (AIDS)
Human leucocyte antigen (HLA) (*Lew-ko-site*)	The subset of Major histocompatibility complex (MHC) genes encoding for cell surface antigen-presenting antigens
Humerus (*Hew-mer-us*)	The largest and longest bone of the upper arm
Humoral immunity (*Hum-or-al*)	The immune response mediated by antibodies, complement proteins, and certain antimicrobial peptides within the extracellular fluid

Key

Primarily associated with anatomy and physiology

Primarily associated with pathophysiology

Term	Definition
Huntington's Disease (HD)	An autosomal dominant, progressive disease of the central nervous system; degeneration of the brain results in uncontrolled movements, emotional problems, and cognitive impairment
Hyaline cartilage (*High-ah-lean kar-til-age*)	Transparent cartilage
Hydatidiform mole (*High-da-tid-e-form*)	Growth of an abnormal fertilised ovum or an overgrowth of placental tissue (during pregnancy)
Hydrocele (*High-dro-seal*)	A collection of serous fluid in the tunica vaginalis surrounding the testis and normally occuring unilaterally
Hydrocephalus (*High-dro-kef-ah-lus*)	Enlargement of the CSF containing cavities, the ventricles, within the brain due to impairment of flow or absorption of the CSF
Hydrolysis (*High-drol-ih-sis*)	When a water molecule is added to a substance which usually splits into two parts
Hydrolytic enzymes (*High-dro-lit-ick*)	Enzymes that catalyse the hydrolysis of a chemical bond
Hydrophilic (*High-dro-fil-ick*)	Having an affinity for water; readily absorbed or dissolved in water
Hydrophobic (*High-dro-fo-bick*)	The tendency to repel or not mix with water
Hydrosalpinx (*High-dro-sal-pinks*)	A distally occluded Fallopian tube filled with serous or clear fluid
Hydrostatic pressure (*High-dro-stat-ick*)	The pressure exerted by the blood against the artery wall by the heart pumping blood at force

Term	Definition
Hydrothorax (*High-dro-tho-racks*)	The collection of serous fluid in the pleural cavity caused by increased hydrostatic pressure or decreased osmotic pressure in blood vessels
Hymen (*High-men*)	A membrane which covers or partly covers the opening of the vagina (until broken by physical activity or intercourse)
Hyperactivation	A state of increased activity or agitation
Hyperaemia (*High-per-e-me-ah*)	Increase in blood supply to an organ
Hyperaldosteronism (*High-per-al-dos-ter-own-ism*)	An excessive secretion of aldosterone that disrupts electrolyte homeostasis, causing an increase in sodium reabsorption in the renal tubule and promoting the loss of potassium and hydrogen. This is often due to aldosterone-secreting adenomas or hyperplasia
Hypercapnia (*High-per-cap-knee-ah*)	Increased levels of carbon dioxide content of the blood
Hypercholesterolaemia (*High-per-kol-es-ter-ol-e-me-ah*)	High levels of cholesterol in the blood
Hyperhomocysteinaemia (*High-per-home-oh-sis-teen-e-me-ah*)	Elevated levels of homocysteine in the blood
Hyperinsulinaemia (*High-per-in-sul-in-e-me-ah*)	High levels of insulin in the blood

Key

Primarily associated with anatomy and physiology

Primarily associated with pathophysiology

Term	Definition
Hypernatraemia (*High-per-na-tree-me-ah*)	High levels of sodium in the blood
Hyperosmolar hyperglycaemic non-ketotic syndrome (HHNKS) (*High-per-oz-mole-ar high-per-gly-see-mick non-key-tot-ick sin-drome*)	A complication of type 2 diabetes mellitus in which hyperglycaemia results in high osmolarity without significant ketoacidosis
Hyperosmolarity (*High-per-oz-mo-lar-it-e*)	The condition of having abnormally high osmolarity
Hyperparathyroidism (*High-per-par-a-thigh-roid-ism*)	Excess amount of parathyroid hormone in the blood
Hyperpituitarism (*High-per-pe-chew-it-ar-ism*)	Increased pituitary secretion
Hyperplasia (*High-per-play-see-ah*)	When cell division multiplies, resulting in increasing number of cells in the organ or tissue affected
Hyperpnoea (*High-per-knee-ah*)	Increase in rate and depth of breathing (normal during exercise)
Hypersensitivity	When the immune response to a substance that is normally harmless is altered, causing damage to cells, tissues and organs (e.g. allergy, autoimmunity)
Hypersomnia (*High-per-som-knee-ah*)	A disorder of sleep characterised by excessive daytime sleepiness, excessive sleep periods and/or the absence of feeling refreshed/reenergised after sleep
Hypersynchronisation (*High-per-sin-crow-nigh-say-shun*)	When numerous neurons in the brain fire excessively from a large electrical impulse generated in one part of the brain, triggering a seizure

Term	Definition
Hypertension (*High-per-ten-shun*)	Persistently elevated blood pressure
Hyperthermia (Pyrexia) (*High-per-ther-me-ah (pie-rex-e-ah)*)	Raised body temperature above 38ºC
Hyperthyroidism (*High-per-thigh-roid-ism*)	When the thyroid gland is overactive and produces too much thyroxine
Hypertonia (*High-per-tone-e-ah*)	High/increased muscle tone
Hypertriglyceridaemia (*High-per-tri-gliss-sir-id-e-me-ah*)	High blood triglyceride levels
Hypertrophic cardiomyopathy (*High-per-tro-fic car-dee-oh-my-op-athy*)	Cardiomyopathy in which hypertrophic changes of the myocardium occur, including of the ventricular septum, without obvious cause, resulting in reduced ability to pump blood effectively
Hypertrophy (*High-per-tro-fee*)	When cells grow in size and increase the size of an organ or tissue. The cells have grown bigger rather than increasing the number
Hyperventilation (*High-per-ven-til-a-shun*)	Ventilation in excess of what is needed for normal elimination of CO_2
Hypervolaemic (*High-per-vol-e-mick*)	Excess volume
Hypo (*High-po*)	Low

Key

Primarily associated with anatomy and physiology

Primarily associated with pathophysiology

Term	Definition
Hypodermis (*High-po-der-miss*)	layer of the skin that connects it to the rest of the body
Hypoglycaemia (*High-po-gly-see-me-ah*)	Low blood sugar
Hypogonadism (*High-po-go-nad-ism*)	*See* Congenital hypogonadotropic hypogonadism (CHH)
Hypoinsulinaemia (*High-po-in-sul-in-e-me-ah*)	Low levels of insulin in the blood
Hypokalaemia (*High-po-cal-e-me-ah*)	Low potassium in the blood
Hypomania (*High-po-main-e-ah*)	When someone is persistently disinhibited and euphoric (but less than with mania)
Hyponatraemia (*High-po-na-tree-me-ah*)	Low sodium in the blood
Hypophosphataemia (*High-po-fos-fa-tae-me-ah*)	Abnormally low level of phosphate in the blood
Hypopituitarism (*High-po-pi-chew-it-ar-ism*)	Decreased pituitary secretion
Hypoplasia (*High-po-play-see-ah*)	Underdevelopment or incomplete development of a tissue or organ
Hypoplastic left heart syndrome (*High-po-plas-tic*)	A syndrome characterised by the left-sided heart structures being underdeveloped and therefore results in a left ventricle that is unable to pump with enough force to meet the needs of the systemic circulation
Hypospadias (*High-po-spay-dee-ahs*)	When the urethral opening is on the underside of the penis
Hypotension (*High-po-ten-shun*)	Low blood pressure

Term	Definition
Hypothalamic-pituitary-adrenal (HPA) axis (*High-po-thal-ah-mick pi-chew-ih-tar-e a-dreen-al*)	A complex neuroendocrine network of relay interactions between the hypothalamus, pituitary gland and adrenal glands that modulate stress responses and other homeostatic processes (e.g. digestion, immune response, and energy regulation)
Hypothalamus (*High-po-thal-amus*)	Several nuclei and tracts of axons in a small area below the thalamus that control the autonomic nervous system, neuroendocrine system, limbic system and management of many crucial functions
Hypothermia (*High-po-ther-me-ah*)	Body temperature below 35ºC
Hypothyroidism (*High-po-thigh-roid-ism*)	When underactivity of the thyroid gland results in insufficient thyroid hormones to meet the needs of the body, causing reduced anabolism and a fall in metabolic rate
Hypotonia (*High-po-tone-e-ah*)	Low/reduced muscle tone
Hypoventilation (*High-po-ven-til-a-shun*)	Decreased ventilation unable to eliminate adequate amounts of CO_2
Hypovolaemia (*High-po-vol-e-me-ah*)	Low blood volume
Hypovolaemic shock (*High-po-vol-e-mick*)	Shock induced by a reduction in circulating blood volume
Hypoxaemia (*High-pox-e-me-ah*)	Decreased levels of oxygen in the blood

Key

Primarily associated with anatomy and physiology

Primarily associated with pathophysiology

Term	Definition
Hypoxia (*High-pox-e-ah*)	Reduction in tissue oxygenation
Hypoxic hypoxia (*High-pox-ick high-pox-e-ah*)	When inadequate amounts of oxygen enter the lungs
Hysteroscopy (*His-ter-oss-ko-pee*)	When the cavity of the uterus is viewed directly through a hysteroscope (a fine telescope)
Iatrogenic (*Eye-a-tro-gen-ick*)	Relating to illness or adverse effect (physical or psychological) caused by healthcare intervention
Ictal phase (*Ick-tal*)	A seizure itself; consists of paroxysmal firing of cerebral neurons
Ictus phase (*Ick-tus*)	*See* Ictal phase
Idiopathic (primary) epilepsy (*Id-e-oh-path-ick*)	Epilepsy for which there is no apparent cause
Idiopathic hypertension	*See* Primary hypertension
Idiosyncratic reactions (*Id-e-oh-sin-kra-tic*)	Serious drug reactions that occur rarely and unpredictably
Ileum (*Ill-e-um*)	Terminal part of the small intestine between the jejunum and the first part of the large intestine – the caecum
Immature chondroblasts (*Kon-dro-blasts*)	Cells that secrete the components of cartilage
Immune complexes	*See* Antigen-antibody complexes
Immune tolerance therapies	Therapies that modify the immune system to prevent it attacking its own body cells in autoimmune disease or foreign cells present in an organ after transplantation

Term	Definition
Immunisation (*Im-une-eye-zay-shun*)	The process of inducing immunity to an infectious organism or agent in an individual or animal through vaccination
Immunodeficiency (*Im-uno-dee-fish-in-see*)	A condition in which the body is unable to produce sufficient antibodies or immunologically sensitised T cells in response to antigens
Immunodeficient (*Im-uno-de-fish-ent*)	Being liable to opportunist infections.
Immunoglobulins (*Im-uno-glob-you-lins*)	Class of proteins that function as antibodies
Immunosuppression (*Im-uno-su-press-shun*)	Partial or complete suppression of the immune response
Immunotherapy (*Im-uno-ther-a-pee*)	The use of agents/drugs to modulate the immune response
Impacted fracture	Fracture where fragments of bone wedge together
Impetigo vulgaris (*Im-pe-tie-go vul-gar-is*)	A common infection of the superficial layers of the epidermis, commonly caused by gram-positive bacteria and is highly contagious. It is characterised by erythematous plaques with a yellow crust that may be itchy or painful to touch
Incretins (*In-kre-tins*)	A group of metabolic hormones released in response to food intake that stimulate a decrease in blood glucose levels by increasing insulin secretion and decreasing glucose production by the liver

Key

Primarily associated with anatomy and physiology

Primarily associated with pathophysiology

Term	Definition
Incubation period (*In-cue-bay-shun*)	The period between introduction of microbe to host and the onset of symptoms of the illness
Independent prescribers (UK)	Health care professionals able to prescribe medicines on their own initiative from the British National Formulary (includes doctors, dentists and some non-medical health professionals, including nurses, pharmacists and, more recently, registered chiropodists, podiatrists, physiotherapists, optometrists and registered therapeutic radiographers)
Induration (*In-dure-a-shun*)	Swelling or hardening of normally soft tissue
Infancy	Period of time from birth to about 24 months
Infarction (*In-farck-shun*)	Tissue death due to inadequate blood supply
Infectious enterocolitis (*En-ter-oh-ko-lie-tis*)	Inflammation of both the small and large intestine due to infection
Infiltration	The diffusion, entry or accumulation of a substance in a tissue or cell
Inflammation	When there is an increased blood supply to a site of injury that triggers an inflammatory response to prevent infection. Second stage of wound healing
Inflammatory bowel disease (IBD)	A group of idiopathic chronic inflammatory disorders of the gastrointestinal tract that includes two major phenotypes, Crohn's disease and ulcerative colitis

Term	Definition
Influenza (*In-flew-en-za*)	A viral infection caused by viruses that belong to the orthomyxoviridae family that can affect both the upper and lower respiratory tract
Ingestion	The taking in of food into the digestive system
Innate immunity (*In-ate*)	The rapid first line of defence against pathogens that responds the same way each time it encounters a pathogen
Inotropes (*Eye-no-tropes*)	Drugs that increase the contractile force of the heart
Insula (*In-su-la*)	Part of the limbic system (insular lobe) that regulates thermosensation, nociception, somatosensation, viscerosensation and gustation
Insulin (*In-su-lin*)	An anabolic hormone which promotes synthesis of proteins, carbohydrates and nucleic acids, reduces blood glucose levels and facilitates entry into the cells of glucose, potassium (K^+), magnesium (Mg^{2+}) and phosphate (PO_4^{3-}). It binds to and activates the appropriate cell membrane receptors causing glucose transporters to promote glucose uptake followed by diverse metabolic events through the body
Insulin growth factors (IGFs)	The most important hormones needed for bone growth during childhood
Intercostal muscles (*In-ter-kos-tal*)	Muscle running along and between the ribs that create and move the chest wall

Key

Primarily associated with anatomy and physiology

Primarily associated with pathophysiology

Term	Definition
Insulin shock (*In-sue-lin*)	A physiological state characterised by excess insulin in the blood, low blood glucose, weakness, and potentially loss of consciousness
Interferons (*In-ter-fear-ons*)	Proteins that prevent viruses replicating
Interleukins (*In-ter-lew-kins*)	A group of cytokines expressed by leucocytes which promote the development and differentiation of T and B lymphocytes and haematopoietic cells
Internal capsule	Major tract of sensory and motor fibres which carry information to and from the cerebral cortex
Internal cervical os	Opening of cervix into the uterus
Internal respiration	The diffusion of gases between blood in the systemic capillaries and the tissues
Interneurons (*In-ter-new-rons*)	Neurons that act as connections between descending and ascending neurons. Also called association neurons
Interphase (*In-ter-phase*)	Stage of cell cycle when growth and preparation for division occur, including duplication of proteins and organelles
Interstitial lung disease (ILD) (*In-ter-sti-chal*)	A group of diffuse parenchymal lung disorders associated with substantial morbidity and mortality
Interstitium (*In-ter-sti-chum*)	An interstitial space within a tissue or organ
Intervertebral discs (*In-ter-ver-te-bral*)	Discs that enable vertebrae to bind together and also function as shock absorbent material
Intestinal obstruction (*In-tess-tin-al*)	Impaired movement of chyme through the intestinal lumen

Term	Definition
Intima (*In-ti-ma*)	Innermost layer of an artery or vein
Intracellular fluid (ICF) (*In-tra-sell-u-lar*)	fluid inside cells in which organelles and other substances are suspended or dissolved
Intracerebral haemorrhage/ haematoma (ICH) (*In-tra-se-re-bral*)	A subset of stroke in which a rupture occurs in a cerebral blood vessel (typically arteries/arterioles) resulting in haemorrhage and haematoma formation in the cerebral parenchyma which can extend into the subarachnoid space
Intracranial hypertension (*In-tra-cray-knee-al*)	The pressure inside the skull, also representing the pressure in brain tissue and cerebrospinal fluid (CSF)
Intracrine (*In-tra-crine*)	Relating to a hormone in which activation of the hormone occurs within the cell where it was created and binds with nuclear receptors to modify function of that cell
Intrinsic (*In-trins-ick*)	Originating within or naturally inherent to the body
Intrinsic AKI	Acute kidney injury (AKI) as a result of abnormalities within the kidney (including damage to the blood vessels, glomeruli and tubules)
Inversion (*In-ver-shun*)	Turning the sole of the foot inwards, outer side of foot on the ground
Ion channels	Pores in the cell membrane that determine the concentration of ions within and outside of the cell

Key

Primarily associated with anatomy and physiology

Primarily associated with pathophysiology

Term	Definition
Iris (*Eye-ris*)	The coloured part of the eye around the pupil that regulates the amount of light entering the eye
Irritable bowel syndrome (IBS)	A gastrointestinal disorder associated with recurrent abdominal pain and altered bowel habits and can be either diarrhoea prevalent or constipation prevalent
Ischaemia (*Iss-key-me-ah*)	A reduction in blood supply to tissue that results in the supply being insufficient
Ischaemic heart disease (*Iss-key-mick*)	*See* Coronary artery disease
Ischaemic hypoxia	When blood supply to tissue is inadequate
Ischaemic stroke	A type of stroke (85% of strokes) secondary to inadequate blood flow to the brain as a result of a partial or complete occlusion of an artery. They can be caused by a thrombus or embolus
Islet cells (*Eye-let*)	Cells of the pancreas that secrete the hormones insulin and glucagon
Isometric contraction (*Eye-zo-met-rick*)	Muscle contraction where there is no change in length of the muscle and no movement but energy is still used
Isotonic contraction (*Eye-zo-ton-ick*)	Muscle contraction where the length of muscle changes enabling body movements and movement of objects
Isovaleric acidaemia (*Eye-zo-val-er-ick a-sid-e-me-ah*)	An autosomal recessive metabolic disorder in which there is impairment of the normal metabolism of the amino acid leucine that leads to acidaemia

Term	Definition
Isthmus (*Is-mus*)	Final section of the aortic arch (the connection between the ascending and descending aorta)
Jaundice (*Jawn-dis*)	Yellow discoloration of the skin and whites of the eyes due to high bilirubin levels
Jejunum (*Jej-ih-num*)	Middle part of the small intestine between the duodenum and ileum
Joint (articulation)	The point at which two or more bones meet
Joint cavity	Cavity filled with synovial fluid secreted by the synovial membrane
Joint effusion (*e-few-shun*)	Presence of increased intra-articular fluid
Junk DNA	Areas of DNA that do not appear to code for any genes
Juxtacrine (*Jux-ta-crine*)	Relating to a hormone which has an effect only on receptors in the immediate neighbourhood of its secretion
Juxtaglomerular apparatus (*Jux-ta-glom-er-u-lar*)	Specialised cells near the glomerulus that stimulate the secretion of the adrenal hormone aldosterone and play a major role in renal autoregulation
Kaposi sarcoma (KS) (*Ca-po-see sar-ko-ma*)	A malignancy of the endothelial cells of blood and lymphatic vessels that initially manifests as a lesion on the skin and mucosal membrane of the mouth

Key

Primarily associated with anatomy and physiology

Primarily associated with pathophysiology

Term	Definition
Karyotype (*Car-e-oh-type*)	The number and appearance of chromosomes in the nucleus
Keratin (*Ker-a-tin*)	A hard, fibrous protein that is found in skin cells and hair
Keratinocytes (*Ker-a-tin-oh-sites*)	Cells that produce keratin
Kernig sign (*Ker-nig*)	Resistance to knee extension in the supine position with the hips and knees flexed against the body
Ketones (*Key-tones*)	Any of a class of organic compounds characterised by a carbonyl group attached to two carbon atoms. They are by-products of the breakdown of fatty acids
Ketonuria (*Key-tone-your-e-ah*)	Excretion of large amounts of ketone bodies in the urine
Krabbe disease	Lysosomal storage disease whereby an enzyme deficiency leads to a lack of myelin and neurodegeneration
Krause end bulbs	General sensory receptors that detect light touch and texture
Kupffer cells (*Cup-fur*)	Macrophages in the sinusoids of the liver that provide a barrier, preventing antigens and bacteria absorbed in the gut returning into the systemic circulation and degrading haemoglobin into haem and globin molecules
Kussmaul respirations (*Coos-mal*)	Laboured, deep breathing often associated with severe metabolic acidosis
Kyphosis (*Ki-pho-sis*)	Excessive convex curvature of the spine
Labia majora (*Lay-bee-ah ma-jor-ah*)	Plump, lip-like structures either side of the vulva

Term	Definition
Labia minora (*Lay-bee-ah min-or-ah*)	Two hairless folds of skin between the labia majora
Labyrinth (*Lab-ih-rinth*)	A series of cavities within the temporal bone that contain the main organs of balance and hearing
Lacrimal (tear) apparatus (*La-kri-mal*)	A system in the eye that is composed of lacrimal glands and ducts that manage the flow of tears
Lacrimal canals	Ducts that carry tears away from the eye
Lacrimal ducts	Ducts that carry tears from the lacrimal gland to the surface of the eye
Lacrimal fluid (tears)	Lubrication for the eye, made by lacrimal glands, containing water, salts, mucus and lysozyme
Lactate (*Lack-tate*)	An ester or salt of lactic acid, the final by-product of anaerobic glycolysis
Lactation (*Lack-tay-shun*)	Production/secretion of breast milk by the mammary glands
Lacteals (*Lack-tea-als*)	Lymphatic vessels of the small intestine
Lactiferous duct (*Lack-tif-er-us*)	Ducts that converge to create a network connecting the nipple to the lobules of the mammary gland and carry breast milk
Lactose intolerance (*Lack-tose*)	The inability to digest lactose
Lacunae (*La-kune-a*)	Cavities in bone created by chondrocytes when they die

Key

Primarily associated with anatomy and physiology

Primarily associated with pathophysiology

Term	Definition
Lamellated corpuscles (*Lam-eh-lay-ted kor-pus-els*)	General sensory receptors that detect deep pressure, stretch, vibration and tickle sensations
Langerhans' cells (*Lang-er-hans*)	Cells that are the first line of defence in the skin and support the immune system by processing antigens
Lanula (*La-nu-la*)	The pale, half-moon shaped area on the nail
Larynx (*La-rinx*)	The hollow, muscular organ that contains the vocal cords and which air passes through in transit to the lungs. Otherwise known as the voice box
Lateral geniculate nucleus (*Jen-ick-you-late new-cle-ass*)	Relay centre in the thalamus for the visual pathway
Legionnaires' disease (*Ley-jon-airs*)	A type of pneumonia caused by *Legionella pneumophila* (gram-negative bacteria) that thrives in warm, moist environments
Leiomyomas (*Lie-oh-my-oh-mas*)	Benign growths derived from smooth muscle and are the commonest type of female reproductive tumours, known as fibroids
Lens (eye)	A curved transparent structure suspended by suspensory ligaments to the ciliary body used to focus light appropriately on the retina
Leptin (*Lep-tin*)	The 'satiety hormone' which regulates how much fat is stored in the body by adjusting the sensation of hunger and the amount of energy expended
Lesion (*Lee-shun*)	An area of abnormal tissue change

Term	Definition
Leucocytes (*Lew-ko-sites*)	White blood cells that provide protection against pathogens. They are mostly found in connective and lymphatic tissue, normally only circulating in the blood for a number of hours
Leucocytosis (*Lew-ko-sigh-toe-sis*)	An increase in the number of leucocytes in the blood
Leukaemias (*Lew-key-me-ahs*)	Malignant disorders of haematopoietic (blood forming) tissue within the bone marrow or peripheral blood supply
Leukopenias (*Lew-ko-pee-knee-ahs*)	Conditions in which there is a reduction in the number of leucocytes
Leukotrienes (*Lew-ko-treens*)	Inflammatory mediators released by mast cells; they are primarily responsible for bronchoconstriction in an asthma attack
Leydig cells (*Lay-dig*)	Cells outside the seminiferous tubules that produce testosterone
Libido (*Li-bee-do*)	The desire for sexual activity
Lichen sclerosus/ Lichen sclerosis (*Li-chin scler-oh-sis/ sus*)	An autoimmune condition in which the vulva is inflamed with areas of very thin epithelium with superficial ulcers due to scratching because of itching
Ligament (*Lig-a-ment*)	A small band of tough, fibrous connective tissue that joins two bones or cartilages or holds together a joint

Key

Primarily associated with anatomy and physiology

Primarily associated with pathophysiology

Term	Definition
Limbic system (*Lim-bick*)	Complex system of neurons and networks in the brain concerned with instinct, mood, emotion and memory
Lipase (*Lie-paze*)	An enzyme that digests fats
Lipogenesis (*Lip-oh-gen-ih-sis*)	The metabolic formation of fat from acetyl-coA and glycerol
Lipolysis (*Lip-ol-ih-sis*)	Breakdown of lipids by hydrolysis to release fatty acids
Lipoma (*Lie-po-ma*)	A benign tumour composed of mature fat cells
Lipophagy (*Lie-poph-a-gee*)	Breakdown and elimination of lipids from cells
Lipopolysaccharides (*Lip-oh-pol-e-sack-a-rides*)	A molecule consisting of combined lipid and polysaccharide
Lipoproteins (*Lip-oh-pro-teens*)	Large molecules which play a central role in the absorption of lipids, and of transporting cholesterol, triglycerides and fat-soluble vitamins through body fluids to and from peripheral tissues and the liver
Lochia (*Losh-e-ah*)	Vaginal discharge lasting approximately 33–60 days postpartum
Locked-in syndrome	A loss of voluntary control of movement, usually from some form of brainstem damage/disorder, but arousability and awareness are retained, that is, the person remains conscious
Long chain fatty acids (LCFA)	A fatty acid with 16 or more carbons

Term	Definition
Low density lipoproteins (LDLs)	Type of lipoprotein largely composed of cholesterol - cells use enzymes to break them down to release the cholesterol
Lumbosacral plexus (*Lum-bo-say-kral*)	Group of neurons extending to the legs
Lumpectomy (*Lump-eck-toe-me*)	Surgical removal of a lump of tissue
Lung compliance	The ease with which the lungs expand
Lupus (*Lew-pus*)	*See* Systemic lupus erythematosus (SLE)
Luteinising hormone (LH) (*Lew-tin-eye-sing*)	A hormone that stimulates Leydig cells to secrete testosterone in men and ovulation and development of the corpus luteum in women
Lymph	The fluid in lymph vessels formed from excess ECF surrounding cells and similar in composition to plasma, with water containing electrolytes, glucose, fats, and leucocytes but normally without erythrocytes and fewer plasma proteins
Lymph node	Small, bean shaped nodes that filter lymph for bacteria, cancer cells, and other potentially harmful substances
Lymphadenopathy (*Lymph-a-den-op-athy*)	Abnormal enlargement of the lymph nodes
Lymphatic system (*Limb-fa-tick*)	System of tubular structures that collect excess ECF and returns it to the systemic circulation
Lymphatic vessels	Tubular structures similar to blood vessels that carry lymph

Key

Primarily associated with anatomy and physiology

Primarily associated with pathophysiology

Term	Definition
Lymphocytes (*Limb-fo-sites*)	Agranulocytes that can destroy cancer cells, cells with a viral infection and foreign cells. There are three types of lymphocytes: B cells, T cells and natural killer (NK) cells
Lymphocytopenia (*Limb-fo-sigh-toe-pee-knee-ah*)	An abnormal reduction in the amount of lymphocytes
Lymphoedema (*Limb-fo-dee-ma*)	Oedema caused by impaired lymphatic drainage of extracellular fluid
Lymphomas (*Limb-fo-mas*)	Cancer of lymphoid tissue
Lymphopenia (*Limb-fo-pee-knee-ah*)	*See* Lymphocytopenia
Lysis (*Lie-sis*)	Deconstruction of a cell by rupture of the cell membrane
Lysosomal enzymes (*Lie-so-zome-al*)	Enzymes that break down macromolecules and bacteria
Lysosome (*Lie-so-zome*)	A cell organelle that contains enzymes which break down unneeded large molecules which are recycled or excreted from the cell
Lysozyme (*Lie-so-zyme*)	A protective bactericidal enzyme
Lytic enzymes (*Li-tick*)	Enzymes that cause lysis
Macrocephaly (*Ma-crow-kef-a-lee*)	When the circumference of the head is larger than expected parameters
Macrocytic (*Ma-crow-sit-ick*)	When a substance is larger in size than normal

Term	Definition
Macrophage (*Ma-crow-phage*)	A form of phagocyte which has a role in both non-specific (innate) and specific (adaptive) defence mechanisms in the body – mature monocyte
Maculae (*Ma-ku-lay*)	Patches of hair and support cells in saccules and utricles of the vestibule. Hair cells are sensory receptors and support cells secrete the otolithic membrane
Maculopapular rash (*Ma-ku-low-pap-you-lar*)	Skin rash characterised by a flat, red area covered with small, confluent bumps
Major histocompatibility complex (MHC) (*His-toe-com-pat-a-bill-it-e*)	Proteins that are recognised as 'self', which in humans are known as the HLA (human leucocyte antigen)
Malabsorption (*Mal-ab-sorb-shun*)	The inability of the intestinal mucosa to absorb digested nutrients
Malabsorption syndromes	Disorders that interfere with intestinal absorptive processes
Malaise (*Mal-aze*)	A feeling of general discomfort, uneasiness or pain
Malignant (*Ma-lig-nant*)	When neoplasms have poorly differentiated, rapid growing cells that are not encapsulated and have the ability to break loose, migrate and form secondary tumours.
Malignant hypertension	A rapid, extreme form of hypertension that can lead to organ damage

Key

Primarily associated with anatomy and physiology

Primarily associated with pathophysiology

Term	Definition
Malnutrition (*Mal-new-tri-shun*)	A lack of nourishment due to inadequate/inappropriate amounts of calories, macronutrients (fat, protein and carbohydrates) and micronutrients (vitamins and minerals). Malnutrition includes undernutrition and overnutrition (excess consumption of nutrients)
Mamillary bodies (*Ma-mill-ar-e*)	Part of the limbic system thought to be a relay center with a distinct role in memory operations
Mammary duct ectasia (*Ma-mar-e duct eck-tay-ze-ah*)	When the lactiferous duct becomes dilated as the duct becomes blocked or clogged and chronic inflammation develops in the surrounding tissues
Maple syrup urine disease	A genetic metabolic disorder affecting the ability to process certain branched-chain amino acids (valine, leucine, isoleucine)
Marfan syndrome (*Mar-fan*)	A connective tissue disorder that results in elongated bones leading to individuals who are tall and thin, with long extremities and digits
Mast cells	Cells that contain basophil granules that release histamine and other inflammatory agents during inflammation and allergic reactions.
Mastectomy (*Ma-stec-toe-me*)	Surgical removal of a breast, including breast tissue, skin and nipple.
Mastitis (*Mass-tie-tis*)	Breast inflammation
Maturation (Remodelling)	Final phase of wound healing that begins during proliferation, whereby adapted fibroblasts attach to collagen fibres and contract to pull the wound margins together (or closer together)

Term	Definition
Meatus (*Me-a-tus*)	A passage or opening leading to the interior of the body
Mechanoreceptors (*Meh-can-oh-re-cep-tors*)	Sensory receptors that respond to mechanical pressure
Medial lemniscal pathways (*Me-dee-al lem-nis-kal*)	Sensory pathways for discriminative touch, vibration and proprioception sensations to the brain
Mediastinum (*Me-dee-a-sty-num*)	The central compartment of the thoracic cavity surrounded by loose connective tissue and contains all the tissues and organs of the chest except the lungs and pleurae
Medulla oblongata (*Meh-dull-ah ob-lon-gata*)	Part of the brain that links with the spinal cord and contains nuclei that act as relay stations for sensory information coming from the spinal cord. Also the location where cortico-spinal and some sensory pathways cross over
Medullary cavity (*Meh-dull-ar-e*)	Cylindrical cavity within the diaphysis containing blood vessels and bone marrow
Megakaryocyte (*Meg-ah-car-e-oh-site*)	A large bone marrow cell responsible for the production of thrombocytes
Meiosis (*My-oh-sis*)	The division that occurs to form the gametes – spermatozoa or ova – in preparation for fertilisation and formation of the zygote which develops into the fetus
Melanin (*Mel-a-lyn*)	A pigment in the skin that protects it from ultraviolet radiation

Key

Primarily associated with anatomy and physiology

Primarily associated with pathophysiology

Term	Definition
Melanocytes (*Mel-a-no-sites*)	Cells that produce melanin
Melatonin (*Mel-a-tone-in*)	Hormone produced by the pineal gland that contributes to the regulation of the sleep-wake cycle
Memory cells	Lymphocytes that have previously encountered specific antigens that on re-exposure to the same antigen rapidly initiate the immune response (memory T cells) or proliferate and produce large amounts of specific antibodies (memory B cells)
Menarche (*Men-are-key or men-are-shay*)	The first occurrence of menstruation
Meninges (*Men-in-gees*)	Three layers of connective tissue that surround the brain and spinal cord
Meningitis (*Men-in-ji-tis*)	Infection and inflammation of the membranes (meninges) and fluid (cerebrospinal fluid) surrounding the brain and spinal cord
Meningocele (*Men-in-jo-seal*)	A protrusion of the meninges through a gap in the spine due to a congenital defect - it contains no neural tissue
Menopause (*Men-oh-pause*)	The ceasing of menstruation
Menorrhagia (*Men-or-ay-gee-ah*)	Excessive menstrual flow
Menstruation (*Men-stru-a-shun*)	Monthly shedding of the endometrium
Merkel cells (*Mer-kel*)	General sensory receptors that detect the tactile sensations of light touch, texture, shapes and edges
Mesenchymal cells (*Me-sen-ki-mal*)	A type of stem cell that develops into vessels (lymphatic and circulatory) and connective tissue

Term	Definition
Messenger RNA (mRNA)	Molecule that carries codes from DNA in the cell nucleus to sites of protein synthesis in ribosomes in cytoplasm. Acts as a template for the polypeptide chain forming a protein
Metabolic acidosis	An acidosis secondary to metabolic production of acid in greater quantities than can be buffered
Metabolic bone disease (*Met-a-bol-ick*)	Disorders of bone metabolism resulting in structural effects on the skeleton
Metabolic rate	Amount of energy used
Metabolic syndrome	A complex syndrome of several pathophysiological conditions marked by obesity, cardiovascular changes and significant insulin resistance
Metabolism (*Meh-tab-oh-lism*)	All of the organic and chemical reactions in the body, using all of the ingested nutrients to create molecules for structure, chemical reactions, and for energy
Metabolites (*Meh-ta-bo-lytes*)	A substance produced during or from taking part in metabolism
Metacarpal bones (*Met-a-car-pal*)	Bones in the middle region of the hand (palm)
Metachromatic leukodystrophy (MLD) (*Met-a-crow-ma-tick lew-ko-dis-tro-fee*)	A lysosomal storage disease
Metaphyses (*Met-a-fis-is*)	The portion of the bone between the diaphysis and the epiphyses

Key

Primarily associated with anatomy and physiology

Primarily associated with pathophysiology

Term	Definition
Metaplasia (*Met-a-play-see-ah*)	When one type of mature cell becomes converted into another which is better able to deal with the conditions causing the change
Metastasis (*Met-a-sta-sis*) (verb, metastasise)	The process whereby cancer cells spread from their original site and proliferate in distant sites
Metastatic spread (*Met-a-sta-tic*)	*See* Metastasis
Metatarsal bones (*Met-a-tar-sal*)	Bones in the region in the middle of the foot
Microbiome (*My-crow-bi-ome*)	The ecological community of commensal, symbiotic and pathogenic microorganisms that coexist within and on the body
Microbiota (*My-crow-bi-oh-ta*)	The microorganisms of a particular location
Microcephaly (*My-crow-kef-a-lee*)	When the circumference of the head is smaller than expected parameters
Microcytic (*My-crow-sit-ick*)	When a substance is smaller in size than normal
Microflora (*My-crow-floor-ah*)	Community of microorganisms (algae, fungi, and bacteria) that live in or on another living organism (e.g. the body)
Microglia (*My-crow-glee-ah*)	Neuroglia that are specialised macrophages capable of phagocytosis, protecting neurons from pathogens
Microorganism (*My-crow-or-gan-ism*)	A microscopic living organism such as a bacterium, virus or fungus
Microvesiculation (*My-crow-ve-sick-u-lay-shun*)	Extracellular vesicles associated with pathophysiological processes

Term	Definition
Microvilli (*My-crow-vill-eye*)	Microscopic cellular membrane projections that increase the surface area of cells. Found on the surface of the small intestine
Micturition (*Mick-ture-ish-un*)	The act of passing urine
Midbrain	Part of the brain that links the thalamus, hypothalamus, pons and medulla oblongata
Migraine (*Mi-grain*)	A severe intermittent disturbance of sensory processing in the CNS that results in a failure in full inhibitory pain control with associated reduction in attentional functional capacity: moderate or severe headache often felt as a throbbing pain on one side of the head
Mineral	Inorganic micronutrient needed for a variety of reasons in the body, largely to do with structure, fluid balance, nervous and muscular activity and blood clotting
Minimally conscious state (MCS)	A disorder of consciousness where a person has a shifting awareness of others and their environment, sometimes responding to some stimuli. Responses are inconsistent but reproducible and indicate that the person is interacting with their environment to some degree
Minute volume	Volume of air/gas inhaled (inhaled minute volume) or exhaled (exhaled minute volume) from a person's lungs in one minute

Key

Primarily associated with anatomy and physiology

Primarily associated with pathophysiology

Term	Definition
Mitochondria (*My-toe-con-dree-ah*)	Cellular organelle known as the 'power house'. ATP is created for storage of energy which is released when required
Mitosis (*My-toe-sis*)	Cell division that results in two genetically identical daughter cells
Mitosis phase	Stage of cell cycle when nuclear division occurs
Mixed urinary incontinence	When stress incontinence and urge incontinence co-exist
Mixture	Molecules of elements and compounds mixed together, without chemical bonds
Molecule	A group of two or more atoms without any electrical charge held together by chemical bonds
Monoclonal antibodies (*Mon-oh-klo-nal*)	Antibodies made in the laboratory to target a specific antigen and numerous copies are produced
Monocytes (*Mon-oh-sites*)	Granulocytes that engulf pathogens and dead neutrophils, clear away debris from dead or damaged cells and present antigens to activate other cells of the immune system
Monoploidy (*Mon-oh-ploy-dee*)	When one member of the chromosome pair is missing
Monosaccharides (*Mon-oh-sack-a-rides*)	Simple carbohydrates (glucose, galactose and fructose) that are easily digested and absorbed in the body
Monosomy (*Mon-oss-oh-me*)	When there is only one copy of a specific chromosome instead of the normal two
Morbidity	The incidence or prevalence of disease

Term	Definition
Morula (*Mor-ooh-la*)	Small bunch of embryonic cells when they enter the uterus (at about three days after fertilisation)
Mosaicism (*Mow-zay-ick-ism*)	Presence of two or more populations of cells with different complement of chromosomes in the same individual.
Motor division/system	Division of the PNS that carries nervous impulses sent from the CNS to cells/ organs/muscles to initiate responses
Motor neuron disease (MND)	A selective and progressive functional loss in upper and lower motor neurons, resulting in impairment or loss of motor function
Movement agnosia (*Ag-no-zee-ah*)	Inability to recognise movement of an object
MRI	Magnetic resonance imaging (MRI) - a type of imaging scan that uses magnetic fields and radio waves to produce detailed images of the inside of the body
mRNA	The template for the polypeptide chain in the formation of a protein
Mucociliary clearance/ escalatory/function (*Mew-ko-sill-e-ar-e*)	The propelling of mucus by cilia from the distal to proximal lung airways
Mucosa (*Mew-ko-za*)	Mucous membrane or a lining of a part of the body that secretes mucus
Mucus (*Mew-kus*)	A viscous slippery secretion produced by mucous membranes. Being rich in mucins, its function is to moisten and protect

Key

Primarily associated with anatomy and physiology

Primarily associated with pathophysiology

Term	Definition
Multifactorial inheritance	The inheritance of a trait as a result of more than one factor, including gene combinations and environmental factors
Multigenic (*Mull-tee-gen-ick*)	Refers to an inherited characteristic specified by a combination of multiple genes
Multiparity (*Mull-tee-par-it-e*)	Having given birth two or more times or having given birth to more than one offspring at a time
Multiple organ dysfunction syndrome (MODS)	When two or more organ systems fail due to the overwhelming uncontrolled inflammatory response
Multiple sclerosis (MS) (*Sclair-oh-sis*)	A chronic, progressive autoimmune disease with multifocal areas of neuronal demyelination disrupting the ability of the nerve to conduct action potentials. It is characterised by chronic inflammation, demyelination, and gliosis (scarring) in the CNS
Muscle	A collection of fibrous tissue that can contract, produce movement or maintain posture
Muscle spindles	General sensory receptors that detect muscle stretch for proprioception
Muscular dystrophies (*Dis-tro-fees*)	A group of genetic disorders that lead to progressive loss of muscle fibres resulting in weakness of voluntary muscles (mostly but not exclusively)
Mutagen (*Mew-ta-jen*)	A chemical or physical agent capable of causing a change in form, quality or other characteristic in a gene thereby causing a mutation
Mutation	When changes in DNA affect the functioning of a gene

Term	Definition
Myalgia (*My-al-gee-ah*)	Muscle pain
Myasthenia gravis (*My-ah-stheen-e-ah gra-vis*)	An autoimmune disorder with an antibody-mediated reaction at the postsynaptic neuromuscular synapse causing muscle weakness
Mycobacterium (*My-co-bac-tear-e-um*) Plural mycobacteria	Non-motile aerobic bacteria that include numerous saprophytes (microorganisms that live on dead/decaying organic matter) and are the pathogens that cause tuberculosis and leprosy
Mycoplasma (*My-co-plaz-mas*)	Microscopic, bacteria-like organism that lacks a cell wall around its cell membrane
Mycoses (*My-co-ses*)	Infection/disease caused by a fungus
Myelin sheath (*My-eh-lin*)	An insulating layer around the axon of a neuron that prevents passive movement of ions across the cell membrane, increasing the speed of conduction of an action potential
Myelomeningocele (*My-eh-low-men-in-gee-oh-seal*)	Neural tissue exposure, resembling a fluid sac adhered to the back. Due to a defect of spine and spinal cord when spine and spinal canal do not close properly. A myelomeningocele is the most serious form of spina bifida
Myenteric plexus (*My-en-ter-ick plex-sus*)	The major nerve supply to the gastrointestinal tract
Myocardial infarction (*My-oh-kar-dee-al in-farc-shun*)	Infarction of the myocardium, normally as a result of occlusion of one or more coronary arteries

Key

Primarily associated with anatomy and physiology

Primarily associated with pathophysiology

Term	Definition
Myocarditis (*My-oh-kar-die-tis*)	Inflammation of the myocardium
Myocardium (*My-oh-kar-dee-um*)	Middle layer of the heart muscle consisting of thin filaments of actin and thick filaments of myosin
Myoclonus (*My-oh-clone-us*)	Brief, sudden, involuntary twitching/jerking of a muscle or a group of muscles
Myocyte (*My-oh-site*)	A contractile cell found in muscle tissue
Myofibrils (*My-oh-phi-brils*)	Small threadlike structures that are the contractile organelles of the skeletal muscle
Myofilaments (*My-oh-phil-a-ments*)	Small protein structures contained within myofibrils
Myoglobin (*My-oh-glow-bin*)	A red coloured, oxygen transmitting protein found only in muscles used to bind oxygen. It consists of one haem molecule with one iron molecule attached to a single globin (protein) chain
Myoglobinuria (*My-oh-glow-bin-your-e-ah*)	Presence of myoglobin in the urine
Myometrium (*My-oh-me-tree-um*)	The smooth muscle tissue forming the middle layer of the uterus
Myotonic muscular dystrophy (MMD) (*My-oh-ton-ick*)	A multisystem disease, caused by genetic mutation, affecting the brain, smooth muscle, skeletal muscle, heart and endocrine systems. It presents with distal muscle weakness, learning difficulties or intellectual disability or both
Myxoedema (*Mix-oh-dee-ma*)	Oedema of the skin and underlying tissues, thickening of the tongue and mucous membranes caused by hypothyroidism, resulting in a waxy appearance and dysarthria

Term	Definition
Narrow complex tachycardia (*Tack-e-kar-dee-ah*)	Tachycardia that originate in the atria
Nasal septum	A thin piece of cartilage and bone inside the nose separating them into the right and left sides (nostrils/nares)
Nasopharynx (*Nase-oh-far-inks*)	Cavity posterior to the nasal cavity and extends to the soft palate
Natriuretic peptide (*Nat-re-ur-ret-ick peptide*)	A peptide that causes natriuresis (renal loss of sodium)
Natural killer cells	Lymphocytes that provide a rapid response to virally infected cells and respond to tumour cell growth
Nausea (*Naw-zee-ah*)	A feeling of sickness and unease with an inclination to vomit
Necrosis (*Neh-crow-sis*)	Death of one or more cells as a result of injury from external stimuli
Negative feedback	Control system in the body that reduces the original stimulus (such as body temperature when it is raised)
Neoplasia (*Knee-oh-play-see-ah*)	Plural of Neoplasm
Neoplasm (*Knee-oh-plasm*)	'New growth' of cells that no longer respond to the body's normal regulatory controls and can be benign or malignant

Key

Primarily associated with anatomy and physiology

Primarily associated with pathophysiology

Term	Definition
Nephrogenic diabetes insipidus (NDI) (*Nef-ro-gen-ick die-a-bee-tees in-sip-id-us*)	A condition when the renal tubule fails to respond to the presence of ADH and is unable to concentrate urine as a result of failure to reabsorb water back into the intravascular space
Nephropathy (*Ne-frop-athy*)	Chronic loss of kidney function
Nephrosclerosis (*Nef-ro-scler-oh-sis*)	Development of sclerotic lesions in the renal arterioles and glomerular capillaries causing them to become thickened and narrowed
Neuralgia (*Neur-al-gee-ah*)	Severe, acute experiences of neuropathic pain that are often repetitive
Neurofibrils (neurofilaments) (*Neu-ro-fib-rills*)	Filaments in neurons that contribute to the transport of cellular material and facilitate axon movement and growth
Neurogenesis (*Neu-ro-gen-ih-sis*)	The process of generating new neurons; growth of new neuronal tissue
Neurogenic bladder (*Neu-ro-gen-ick*)	Bladder dysfunction secondary to impaired nervous control
Neurogenic bowel (*Neu-ro-gen-ick*)	Colon dysfunction secondary to impaired nervous control
Neurogenic shock (*Neu-ro-gen-ick*)	A type of shock secondary to disruption of the autonomic pathways within the spinal cord that results in a triad of hypotension, bradycardia and hypothermia
Neuroglia (*Neu-ro-glee-ah*)	Non-neuronal cells that support and protect neurons

Term	Definition
Neuromuscular junction (*Neu-ro-mus-cu-lar*)	The synapse between a motor neuron and skeletal muscle fibre separated by a synaptic cleft
Neuron (nerve cell) (*Neu-ron*)	Specialised cell of the nervous system that transmits nervous impulses (action potentials)
Neuronal plasticity/ neuroplasticity (*Neu-ro-nal plaz-tis-it-e*)	The ability of the nervous system to create and reorganise synaptic connections in response to early development, learning, experience or following injury
Neuropathy (*Neu-rop-athy*)	Disease or dysfunction of one or more peripheral nerves, typically causing numbness or weakness
Neurotoxins (*Neu-ro-tox-ins*)	Endotoxins that inhibit the release of neurotransmitters
Neurotransmitter (*Neu-ro-trans-mit-er*)	Chemical messenger that transmits nerve signals across a synapse
Neutropenia (*Neu-tro-peen-e-ah*)	A fall in production or an increase in loss from the blood of neutrophils
Neutrophils (*Neu-tro-fils*)	Granulocytes that engulf bacteria and cellular debris or use chemical agents (lysozyme and peroxidase) to destroy foreign bodies
Niemann–Pick disease	A genetic disease that affects lipid metabolism
Nitric oxide (NO) (*Nigh-tric ox-ide*)	A gas that causes and maintains vasodilation and contributes to increased vascular permeability

Key

Primarily associated with anatomy and physiology

Primarily associated with pathophysiology

Term	Definition
NMDA receptor antagonists	A class of anaesthetics that work to antagonise/inhibit the action of the N-methyl-D-aspartate receptor (NMDAR)
Nociception (*No-see-sep-shun*)	Perception of pain
Nociceptors (*No-see-sep-tors*)	Sensory receptors that respond to pain stimuli
Nodes of Ranvier (*Nodes of Ran-ve-ey*)	Gaps between areas of myelination on the axon where ions can easily flow into the ECF
Non-cicatricial (*Non-sick-a-trish-al*)	Non-scarring
Non-communicable disorders/disease	Disease not contracted by contact but occurring as a result of a range of risk factors or occurrences (e.g. trauma, poor diet)
Non-neoplastic epithelial disorders (*Knee-oh-plazz-tick ep-e-thee-lee-al*)	Refers to a number of disorders which can affect the vulval epithelium
Normocytic (*Nor-mo-sit-ick*)	When a substance is the size expected
N-terminal pro b-type natriuretic peptide (NT-proBNP)	A polypeptide released by the ventricles of the heart in response to excessive stretching of the heart. Can be used to diagnose heart failure
Nuchal (*Neu-cal*)	Relating to the nape of the neck
Nuclei (*Neu-klee-eye*)	Brain structures composed of compact clusters of neurons
Nucleolus (*Neu-klee-oh-lus*)	Contained within the nucleus of the cell, this structure is involved in the formation of ribosomes

Term	Definition
Nucleus (*Neu-klee-us*)	Cellular organelle that contains the genetic information (DNA) within chromosomes. It provides the template (RNA) for protein formation
Nutrient foramina (*For-a-mean-a*)	The external opening for the entrance of blood vessels in a bone
Nutrients	Substances that are ingested, digested, absorbed and metabolised to maintain homeostasis through their roles in structure and function within the body, primarily carbohydrates, proteins, fats, minerals and vitamins
Nutrition	Food or nourishment. Also the branch of science that deals with nutrients and nutrition; the scientific foundation for dietetics
Nystagmus (*Nigh-stag-mus*)	Rapid involuntary movements of the eyes
Obesity	Abnormal or excessive fat accumulation that may impair health
Obligate aerobes (*Ob-li-gate air-robes*)	Microorganisms that can only grow in the presence of oxygen
Oblique fracture	Fracture at an angle through the bone
Obstructive shock	A form of shock that occurs as a result of an obstruction in blood circulation
Oedema (*Oh-dee-ma*)	The observable accumulation of excess interstitial fluid secondary to an imbalance between capillary filtration and lymph drainage

Key

Primarily associated with anatomy and physiology

Primarily associated with pathophysiology

Term	Definition
Oesophageal varices (*Oh-sof-a-gee-al var-ih-sees*)	Dilated submucosal veins in the lower oesophagus secondary to portal hypertension
Oesophagus (*Oh-sof-a-gus*)	A muscular tube that connects the oropharynx to the stomach, passing through the diaphragm
Oestrogen (*E-stro-jen*)	Any of several steroid hormones, largely secreted by the ovaries and placenta
Oestrogens (*E-stro-jens*)	Refers to the group of oestrogenic hormones (e.g. oestradiol and oestrogen), classically referred to as female sex hormones although some are present in men in lesser amounts. They are associated with development of secondary sexual characteristics, growth and maturation of long bones, sexual function and menstruation
Olfaction (*Ol-fac-shun*)	Sense of smell
Olfactory epithelium (*Ol-fac-tory ep-e-thee-lee-um*)	Specialised tissue inside the nasal cavity involved in smell
Olfactory glands	Glands in the olfactory mucosa that produce mucus to lubricate the surface of the olfactory epithelium
Olfactory mucosa	Found within the nasal cavity, this section of the nasal mucosa contains the sensory nerve endings for smell
Oligoclonal bands	Bands of immunoglobulins suggesting inflammation of the central nervous system due to infection or another disease
Oligodendrocytes (*Ol-ih-go-den-dro-sites*)	A type of neuroglial cell that produces myelin in the central nervous system

Term	Definition
Oligohydramnios (*Ol-ih-go-high-dram-knee-ohz*)	Reduced amniotic fluid
Oligomenorrhea (*Ol-ih-go-men-or-e-ah*)	Infrequent or very light menstruation
Oligosaccharides (*Ol-ih-go-sack-a-rides*)	Carbohydrates composed of approximately three to nine monosaccharides and used to make glycoproteins and glycolipids
Oligozoospermia (*Ol-ih-go-zoo-sperm-e-ah*)	Low sperm count
Oliguria (*Ol-ih-go-your-e-ah*)	Urine output that is less than 1 ml/kg/h in infants, less than 0.5 ml/kg/h in children, and less than 400 ml or 500 ml per 24h in adults
Omentum (*Oh-men-tum*)	A fold of visceral peritoneal tissue that hangs from the stomach
Oncogenes (*On-ko-jeans*)	A mutated gene that may cause the growth of cancer cells
Oogenesis (*Ooh-jen-ih-sis*)	The process of female gamete formation
Ophthalmoplegia (*Op-thal-mo-plee-gee-ah*)	Paralysis or weakness of the eye muscles
Opportunists	Microbes which are normally harmless within the body but can cause disease when the body is immunocompromised
Opsonisation (*Op-son-eye-say-shun*)	The process by which a pathogen is marked for destruction by phagocytosis

Key

Primarily associated with anatomy and physiology

Primarily associated with pathophysiology

Term	Definition
Optic chiasm (*Op-tick kai-asm*)	Point on the visual nerve pathways where half the fibres go to the lateral geniculate nucleus on the same side of the brain the and the other half cross over to the opposite side
Optic disc	A convergence of the retinal ganglion cells to form the optic nerve
Orchidopexy (*Or-kid-o-pex-e*)	Surgical treatment of undescended testis
Organ	A differentiated structure with specific function(s) made up of organised cells and tissues
Organ of Corti	Structure in the cochlea that converts sound vibrations into nervous impulses through the long, stiff hairs called stereocilia
Organelle (*Or-gan-el*)	A cellular structure with a specific function (small cell organ)
Organomegaly (*Or-gan-oh-meg-a-lee*)	Abnormal enlargement of an organ
Orgasm (*Or-gaz-im*)	The pleasurable, whole body sensation that makes sexual experiences attractive to people
Oropharynx (*Oro-far-inks*)	The part of the pharynx below the soft palate and above the epiglottis that is continuous with the mouth. This cavity extends from the soft palate to the epiglottis
Orthopnoea (*Orth-op-knee-ah*)	Difficulty in breathing when lying flat
Oscillation (*Oss-ih-lay-shun*)	Regular fluctuation or vibration about a central point
Osmolality (*Oss-mo-lal-it-e*)	The concentration of osmotically active particles per kilogram of solvent

Term	Definition
Osmolarity (*Oss-mo-lar-it-e*)	The concentration of osmotically active particles per 1000ml of solution
Osmoreceptors (*Oss-mo-re-cept-ors*)	A group of specialised sensory neurons in the hypothalamus that are stimulated by increased osmolality of the extracellular fluid
Osmosis (*Oss-mo-sis*)	The movement of water across a semipermeable membrane from a dilute/hypotonic solution (with low osmotic pressure) to a more concentrated/hypertonic solution (which has a higher osmotic pressure)
Osmotic diuresis (*Oss-mot-ick die-yur-e-sis*)	Excess urine production as a result of osmotic particles being excreted by the kidney, carrying water with them
Osmotic pressure	The pressure exerted by plasma proteins and some electrolytes in the plasma inside the capillaries, pulling water and small molecules towards them. Includes the pressure exerted in pulling water across a semipermeable membrane
Ossicles (*Oss-ick-ills*)	Tiny bones in the ear that connect with the eardrum, transferring and magnifying sound vibration from the auditory canal to the inner ear
Ossification (*Oss-if-ick-a-shun*)	The formation of bone
Osteitis deformans (*Oss-tee-eye-tis def-or-mans*)	*See* Paget disease of bone (PDB)

Key

Primarily associated with anatomy and physiology

Primarily associated with pathophysiology

Term	Definition
Osteoarthritis (*Oss-tee-oh-ar-thry-tis*)	Joint disease characterised by the loss of and damage to articular cartilage, inflammation, osteophytosis (formation of bone spurs) and thickening of subchondral bone
Osteoblasts (*Oss-tee-oh-blasts*)	Bone building cells that synthesise and secrete collagen fibres and other organic components and also initiate calcification of bone matrix
Osteoclasts (*Oss-tee-oh-clasts*)	Bone cells formed from fused monocytes that secrete powerful lysosomal enzymes and acids for dissolving the protein and mineral matrix
Osteocytes (*Oss-tee-oh-sites*)	Bones cells, derived from osteoblasts, found in mature bone and are the main cell type in bone
Osteogenesis (ossification) (*Oss-tee-oh-jen-ih-sis (oss-if-ick-a-shun)*)	Formation of bone
Osteogenic (*Oss-tee-oh-jen-ick*)	Bone producing
Osteogenic cells	Bone cells derived from mesenchymal cells (adult stem cells) that develop into osteoblasts
Osteomalacia (*Oss-tee-oh-mal-a-see-ah*)	Softening of bones due to the inadequate and slowed mineralisation of osteoid in mature bone
Osteomyelitis (*Oss-tee-oh-my-eh-lie-tis*)	Infection of bone
Osteon (*Oss-tee-on*)	Chief structural unit of compact bone
Osteopenia (*Oss-tee-oh-pee-knee-ah*)	A reduction in bone density greater than would be expected for age

Term	Definition
Osteophytosis (*Oss-tee-oh-fi-toe-sis*)	New bone formation of joint margins leading to osteophytes (bone spurs)
Osteoporosis (*Oss-tee-oh-po-ro-sis*)	A complex, chronic, progressive metabolic bone disease, multifactorial in nature, characterised by a decrease in bone mineral density (BMD) leading to an increased risk of fractures
Otalgia (*Ot-al-gee-ah*)	Ear pain
Otitis media (*Oh-tie-tis me-dee-ah*)	Inflammation of the middle ear
Otolithic membrane (*Ot-oh-lith-ick*)	A thick gelatinous glycoprotein layer in the vestibule that detects movement through gravitational pull
Ova (*Oh-va*)	*See* Ovum
Overactive bladder syndrome	A syndrome characterised by increased urinary frequency, nocturia and urgency with or without urge incontinence in the absence of infection
Overflow incontinence	The involuntary loss of urine due to bladder distension in the absence of detrusor muscle activity
Overweight	*See* Obesity
Oviduct (*Oh-vee-duct*)	*See* Fallopian tube
Ovulation (*Ov-you-lay-shun*)	A component of the menstrual cycle whereby a mature ovarian follicle releases an ovum (female gamete) which moves down the fallopian tube towards the uterus

Key

Primarily associated with anatomy and physiology

Primarily associated with pathophysiology

Term	Definition
Ovum (*Oh-vum*) Plural ova	The female gamete
Oxidation (*Ox-ih-day-shun*)	The loss of electrons or an increase in oxidation state by a molecule, atom, or ion
Oxidative phosphorylation (*Ox-ih-day-tiv fos-for-ih-lay-shun*)	The synthesis of ATP by phosphorylation of ADP
Oxidative stress (*Ox-ih-day-tiv*)	An imbalance between the production of free radicals and the ability of the body to counteract or detoxify their harmful effects through neutralisation by antioxidants
Oxytocinergic (*Ox-e-toe-sin-er-gic*)	Releasing or involving oxytocin
Paget disease of bone (PDB)	A progressive bone disease where there is an increased rate of metabolic activity in bone leading to localised, abnormal and excessive remodelling of bone
Palpebrae (*Pal-pe-bray*)	The eyelids
Palpebral fissure (*Pal-pe-bra-l*)	The gap between open eyelids
Panacinar (*Pan-a-sin-ar*)	Involves the acini at the terminal alveoli
Pancreatic exocrine insufficiency (*Pan-kre-at-ick ex-oh-crine*)	The inability to produce pancreatic enzymes
Pancreatic juice (*Pan-kre-at-ick*)	An alkaline liquid secreted by the pancreas containing sodium bicarbonate, inactive proteolytic enzymes and a number of active enzymes

Term	Definition
Pancreatitis (*Pan-kre-a-tie-tis*)	Inflammation of the pancreas
Pandemic (*Pan-dem-ick*)	A condition which spreads across a large region or worldwide
Paneth cells (*Pan-eth*)	Endocrine cells in the crypts of the epithelium
Pannus (*Pan-us*)	A thickened layer of fibrovascular tissue or granulation tissue
Papanicolaou (Pap) smear (test) (*Pa-pa-nick-oh-lau*)	Procedure in which cells are retrieved from the cervix using a spatula in order to examine them for changes that may indicate cancer or other disease processes
Papillary layer (*Pa-pil-ar-e*)	Upper layer of the dermis made up of fine and loosely arranged collagen fibres that interweave with the epidermis
Papilloedema (*Pa-pil-oh-dee-ma*)	Oedema of the optic disc
Papules (*Pa-pules*)	A solid elevation of skin with distinct margins and no visible fluid
Paracellularly (*Par-a-sell-you-lar-lee*)	Refers to movement/transport of substances between cells.
Paracrine (*Par-a-crine*)	Relating to a hormone which has an effect only in the neighbourhood of its secretion
Paraesthesia (*Para-es-these-e-ah*)	Abnormal sensations such as numbness, tingling, or burning
Parahippocampal gyrus (*Par-a-hip-oh-camp-al*)	Structure of the limbic system that works with the hippocampus in processing declarative memory

Key

Primarily associated with anatomy and physiology

Primarily associated with pathophysiology

Term	Definition
Paraneoplastic syndromes (*Par-a-knee-oh-plas-tick*)	Disorders that are triggered by an altered immune system response to a neoplasm
Paraphimosis (*Par-a-fim-oh-sis*)	When the foreskin becomes trapped behind the corona of the glans penis, compromising arterial supply to the gland and preventing venous and lymphatic return
Paraplegia (*Par-a-ple-gee-ah*)	Injury to the thoracic, lumbar, or sacral regions of the spinal cord, including the cauda equina and conus medullaris resulting in loss of function of the lower body
Parasite (*Par-a-site*)	An organism which lives in or on another organism (known as the host) and benefits by deriving nutrients from the host but provides no benefit to the host
Parasympathetic nervous system (*Par-a-sim-pa-thet-ick*)	A division of the autonomic nervous system which reduces the activity of many of the systems of the body, but increases digestion, absorption and storage of nutrients
Parenteral (*Par-en-ter-al*)	Referring to a route of entry of a substance other than through the enteral route
Parkinson's/ Parkinson's disease	A progressive neurodegenerative disorder associated with decreased dopamine in parts of the brain, largely due to destruction of the nigrostriatal neurons (in the basal ganglia) that results in loss of smooth, coordinated movement

Term	Definition
Passive diffusion	The passive movement of a solute from an area of high concentration to an area of lower concentration until the concentration of the solute is uniform throughout and reaches equilibrium
Patella (*Pa-tell-ah*)	A small triangular bone found at the front of the knee joint (kneecap)
Patent ductus arteriosus (PDA) (*Pay-tent duct-us ar-tear-e-oh-sus*)	When the fetal ductus arteriosus remains patent after birth
Pathogen (*Path-oh-gen*)	An agent causing disease or illness to its host
Pathogenesis (*Path-oh-gen-eh-sis*)	The biological processes that lead to development of a disease
Pathogenic (*Path-oh-gen-ick*)	Ability to cause or produce disease
Pelvic girdle (*Gur-dil*)	Unit of two pelvic bones (hip bones)
Pelvic inflammatory disease (PID)	Infection of the upper female genital tract including the uterus, ovaries, fallopian tubes, and cervix
Penetrance (*Pen-eh-trance*)	The extent that the trait carried in the abnormal gene presents the disorder
Penumbra (*Pen-um-bra*)	An area of ischaemic tissue in which infarction is evolving but is reversible if circulation/perfusion is restored

Key

Primarily associated with anatomy and physiology

Primarily associated with pathophysiology

Term	Definition
Pepsinogen (*Pep-sin-oh-gen*)	A proenzyme produced by chief cells in the stomach and converted to its active form, pepsin, for digestion of protein
Peptic ulcer disease	Ulceration that occurs in the gastric or intestinal mucosal lining
Perforation	When erosion, infection, or other factors produce a weak point in an organ or structure that can rupture as a result of internal pressure
Perfuse	To move fluid and nutrients through to cells of organs/tissues
Perfusion	The delivery of blood to the capillary bed in systemic circulation. Also refers to the amount of blood perfusing the capillaries around the alveoli
Pericardium (*Per-e-kar-dee-um*)	Outermost layer of the heart muscle composed of two sacs which cover the outside of the heart – the parietal pericardium and visceral pericardium (or epicardium)
Perichondrium (*Per-e-con-dree-um*)	Dense, irregular connective tissue which surrounds most cartilage, containing blood vessels and nerves
Perilymph (*Per-e-lim-ph*)	Fluid within the scala tympani and scala vestibule
Perineum (*Per-e-knee-um*)	Area between the anus and the scrotum or vulva
Periosteum (*Per-e-oss-tee-um*)	The tough connective tissue membrane that covers the outside of the bone (except where there is articular cartilage)
Peripartum cardiomyopathy (*Per-i-par-tum kar-dee-oh-my-op-athy*)	Cardiomyopathy that develops in the last month of pregnancy or up to five months after delivery

Term	Definition
Peripheral artery disease	A circulatory disorder caused by the build-up of plaque in the major arteries that supply the legs, arms and pelvis
Peripheral nerve disorders	Disorders involving motor and/or sensory neurons of the peripheral nervous system resulting in muscle weakness and/or atrophy and possibly sensory changes
Peripheral nervous system (PNS)	All of the nervous system outside the central nervous system
Peripheral resistance	The resistance to the flow of blood from the wall of the arterial vessels
Peristalsis (*Per-e-stal-sis*)	The ripple like waves created by the relaxation and contraction of muscle in a tubular structure that results in the movement of material along its length
Peritoneum (*Per-it-oh-knee-um*)	The serosa of the small and large intestine composed of two serous membranes – the parietal, lining the walls of the abdomen, and visceral, covering the abdominal organs
Pernicious anaemia (*Per-nish-us a-knee-me-ah*)	Deficiency in the production of erythrocytes through a lack of vitamin B_{12}
Perseveration (*Per-sev-er-a-shun*)	Persistence of a single thought
Petechial rash (*Pe-tea-key-al*)	Pinpoint, round spots on the skin secondary to microhaemorrhages

Key

Primarily associated with anatomy and physiology

Primarily associated with pathophysiology

Term	Definition
Peyer's patches (*Pay-ers*)	Aggregations of lymph tissue within the lower part of the ileum
pH	A chemical term which indicates the level of acidity/alkalinity in a solution and is determined by the amount of hydrogen ions (H⁺) in a solution
Phaeochromocytoma (*Fay-oh-chrome-oh-sigh-toe-ma*)	A neuroendocrine tumour of the adrenal medulla that secretes high amounts of catecholamines
Phagocytes (*Fay-go-sites*)	Mobile white cells which engulf and destroy pathogens
Phagocytosis (*Fay-go-sigh-toe-sis*)	Process by which a cell (e.g. white blood cell) engulfs a pathogen, other cells, cell debris or foreign particles (verb phagocytose)
Phalanges (*Fa-lan-gees*)	Bones of the digits of the hand and feet
Pharmacodynamics (*Far-ma-ko-die-na-micks*)	The study of how drugs affect the body
Pharmacokinetics (*Far-ma-ko-kin-et-icks*)	The study of the physiological absorption, distribution, metabolism, and excretion of drugs within the body
Pharmacology (*Far-ma-col-oh-gee*)	The study of drugs including their origin, composition, pharmacokinetics, therapeutic use, and toxicology
Pharyngitis (*Far-in-ji-tis*)	Inflammation of the pharynx
Pharynx (*Far-inks*)	The section of the gastrointestinal tract that extends from the mouth and nasal cavities to the larynx
Phenotype (*Fee-no-type*)	The observable expression of an individual's characteristics resulting from the interaction of its genotype with the environment

Term	Definition
Phenylalanine (*Fe-nil-al-ah-neen*)	An essential amino acid that is metabolised to tyrosine
Phenylketonuria (*Fe-nil-key-tone-you-ree-ah*)	A genetic disorder whereby the amino acid phenylalanine builds up in the body as a result of a defect in the gene that helps create the enzyme needed to break it down. Can cause intellectual disability, seizures, behavioural problems and mental disorders
Phimosis (*Fim-oh-sis*)	An inability to retract the foreskin over the glans penis
Phlebitis (*Fle-bi-tis*)	Inflammation of the walls of a vein
Phospholipids (*Fos-fo-lip-ids*)	Type of fats composed of one glycerol molecule, two fatty acids, and a phosphate group
Photoaging	Ageing of the skin as a result of sun exposure and pigmentation
Photoreceptors	Sensory receptors that respond to light as a stimulus
Photosensitivity	Sensitivity to light or ultraviolet radiation
Pia mater (*Pee-ah*)	A thin, impermeable fibrous membrane adjacent to the brain and spinal cord ensuring that CSF remains within the subarachnoid space. Blood vessels pass through the pia mater to the brain and spinal cord
Pili (*Pill-eye*)	Structures on the surface of bacteria that enable them to attach to a host cell

Key

Primarily associated with anatomy and physiology

Primarily associated with pathophysiology

Term	Definition
Piloerection (*Pil-oh-e-reck-shun*)	Involuntary erection of hairs on the skin due to a sympathetic reflex
Pineal gland (*Pin-e-al*)	Gland that secretes serotonin during the day and melatonin at night, in regulating the sleep–wake cycle
Pinna (*Pin-ah*)	*See* Auricle
Pituitary gland (*Pi-tui-it-ar-e*)	A small pea-sized extension below the hypothalamus that links the nervous and endocrine systems
Pituitary stalk	The connection between the hypothalamus and the posterior pituitary
Placenta (*Pla-cent-ah*)	The vascular organ formed in the uterus during pregnancy from maternal and embryonic tissues to deliver oxygen and nutrients to the fetus and move fetal waste products into the maternal circulation
Placenta abruptio/ placental abruption (*Pla-cent-ah a-brup-tee-oh/Pla-cent-al a-brup-shun*)	When the placenta comes away from the lining of the uterus before delivery of the baby occurs, most commonly at around 25 weeks of gestation
Placenta praevia (*Pla-cent-ah pre-v-e-ah*)	When the placenta has implanted in the lower part of the uterus or over the cervix
Plaque (*Plack*)	An accumulation of semi-solid substances on the surface of tissue (e.g. within an artery or on the surface of a tooth)
Plantar flexion (*Plan-tar*)	Movement that lowers the foot (points the toes)

Term	Definition
Plasma (*Plaz-ma*)	The colourless fluid part of blood or lymph in which cells are suspended, primarily composed of water and plasma proteins, enzymes, hormones, gases, electrolytes, and waste products
Plasmids (*Plaz-mids*)	Pieces of DNA that replicate independently from the host's chromosomal DNA
Plasticity (*Plas-tis-it-e*)	The adaptability of an organism to changes in its environment or differences between its various habitats
Platelet-activating factor (PAF)	A pro-inflammatory lipid molecule that activates neutrophils through chemotaxis and causes platelet aggregation and degranulation, inflammation, and anaphylaxis
Pleural cavity (*Plu-ral*)	Thin, fluid filled space between the two layers of the pleural membrane
Pleural effusion (*Plu-ral e-fuse-shun*)	An abnormal collection of fluid in the pleural cavity
Pleural membrane	The serous membrane lining the lungs
Plicae (*Pli-kay*)	A fold or ridge of tissue
Pluripotent (*Plur-e-po-tent*)	The ability of a cell to differentiate into any type of cell or tissue but not a complete organism
Pneumonia (*New-moan-e-ah*)	Inflammatory condition of the lungs, primarily alveoli and bronchioles

Key

Primarily associated with anatomy and physiology

Primarily associated with pathophysiology

Term	Definition
Pneumotaxic centre (*New-mo-tax-ick*)	Area in the upper pons responsible for regulating ventilation (with the apneustic centre)
Pneumothorax (*New-mo-thor-axe*)	The presence of air in the pleural cavity caused by rupture of either the parietal or visceral pleura
Polycystic ovary syndrome (PCOS) (*Pol-e-sis-tick*)	A disorder involving infrequent, irregular or prolonged menstrual periods, anovulation and often excessive androgen levels
Polycythaemia (*Pol-e-sigh-theme-e-ah*)	A condition in which there is a raised level of red blood cells (erythrocytes) or haemoglobin
Polycythaemia vera (*Pol-e-sigh-theme-e-ah vera*)	A malignant disorder of haematopoietic stem cells leading to raised amounts of erythrocytes
Polydipsia (*Pol-e-dip-see-ah*)	Excessive thirst
Polygenic inheritance (*Pol-e-gen-ick*)	The inheritance of a single trait (phenotype) that is controlled by two or more different genes
Polyhydramnios (*Pol-e-high-dram-knee-os*)	Increased amniotic fluid
Polymicrobial (*Pol-e-my-crow-bee-al*)	Polymicrobial diseases are caused by combinations of viruses, bacteria, fungi, and parasites which together cause more severe diseases
Polymorphic (*Pol-e-mor-fick*)	Occurring in more than one form
Polymorphism (*Pol-e-mor-fizz-em*)	The manifestation of two or more genetically determined phenotypes in a certain population
Polypeptides (*Pol-e-pep-tides*)	Amino acids combined together by peptide bonds

Term	Definition
Polyphagia (*Pol-e-fage-e-ah*)	Excessive hunger
Polyploidy (*Pol-e-ploy-dee*)	When a cell contains more than two paired (homologous) sets of chromosomes
Polysaccharides (*Pol-e-sack-a-rides*)	Carbohydrates composed of many monosaccharides, usually more than ten, and are often used as a form of energy storage, such as glycogen in the liver and muscle cells
Polyuria (*Pol-e-your-e-ah*)	An excessive amount of urine production
Pons	Collection of nerve fibres connecting the two hemispheres of the cerebellum, brain and the spinal cord. It also acts as a relay station, contains cranial nuclei and has a role in regulating breathing
Porphyria (*Por-fi-re-ah*)	A genetic disorder where there is impairment in the ability to produce haem, resulting in increased formation and excretion of chemicals called porphyrins
Portal fissure (*Por-tal fish-ur*)	Fissure in the liver that allows for entry and exit of blood vessels, lymph vessels, nerves and bile ducts
Portal hypertension	High pressure in the hepatic portal vein
Portal vein	Vein that delivers nutrient rich deoxygenated blood from the stomach, pancreas and small and large intestine to the liver

Key

Primarily associated with anatomy and physiology

Primarily associated with pathophysiology

Term	Definition
Positive feedback	Control system that enhances the original stimulus (such as blood clotting)
Posterior cord syndrome	Damage to the posterior third of the spinal cord or the posterior spinal artery, leading to loss of light touch, vibration, and proprioception sensations
Post-ictal phase (*Post-ick-tal*)	Period after a seizure with temporary neurological dysfunction
Postpartum (*Post-par-tum*)	The period immediately after birth of a child (six weeks normally)
Postpartum haemorrhage (PPH)	The loss of 500ml of blood within 24 hours of delivery
Postrenal AKI	Acute kidney injury (AKI) secondary to an obstruction in the urinary collection system
Post-traumatic epilepsy (PTE)	A recurrent seizure disorder occurring due to traumatic brain injury
Prebiotic (*Pre-bye-ot-ick*)	An ingested substance not digested in the small intestine that beneficially affects the host by selectively stimulating the growth and/or activity of one or a limited number of bacteria that can improve the host's health
Pre-eclampsia (*Pre-e-clam-see-ah*)	A disorder of pregnancy characterised by the onset of hypertension and (often) proteinuria
Prefrontal cortex	An area of grey matter in the anterior frontal lobe involved in the complex regulation of cognition, emotion, and behavioural function
Preputial orifice (*Pre-pew-shal*)	Opening of the foreskin
Pressure ulcers	*See* Decubitus ulcer

Term	Definition
Priapism (*Pry-a-pism*)	Prolonged erection of the penis that is non-sexual
Primary adrenal cortical insufficiency	When there is insufficient production of the hormone cortisol from the adrenal cortex. There may also be insufficient aldosterone production
Primary encephalitis	When a pathogen directly infects the brain and spinal cord
Primary hypertension	When blood pressure is elevated without evidence of another disease causing it
Primary immunodeficiency	Disorder as a result of a single gene mutation that results in immune dysregulation, autoimmunity and recurrent infection
Primary injury (neurological)	Referring to damage that occurs at the time of trauma, i.e. the physical effect of mechanical forces on the brain or spinal cord
Primary intention	Uncomplicated healing of the skin where wound edges are joined together and there is no tissue deficit to remedy
Primary polydipsia	An excessive intake of water that suppresses the secretion of ADH
Probiotics	Live microorganisms which confer a health benefit on the host.
Procallus (*Pro-kal-us*)	Granulation tissue formed at the site of fracture

Key

Primarily associated with anatomy and physiology

Primarily associated with pathophysiology

Term	Definition
Procarboxypeptidase (*Pro-kar-box-e-pep-tid-aze*)	The inactive precursor of carboxypeptidase
Processus vaginalis (*Pro-ses-us va-gin-ah-lis*)	The peritoneal tunnel through which the testes migrate from the retroperitoneum toward the scrotum during embryological development
Prodromal (*Pro-drow-mal*)	Phase that precedes a seizure involving symptoms and signs including insomnia, headache, reduced tolerance threshold, increased agitation, low mood, and emotional lability. Also refers to the short time of generalised/mild symptoms (malaise, muscle aches) that precede illness
Progression	Developing or moving gradually towards a more advanced state. For example, when a mutant dividing cell begins to exhibit malignant properties
Prokaryotes (*Pro-car-e-oats*)	A single-celled organism without a distinct nucleus with a membrane and specialised organelles
Proliferation (*Pro-lif-er-a-shun*)	Rapid reproduction of a cell, part, or organism
Proliferation (phase)	Stage of wound healing that involves angiogenesis and production of new structural tissue that begins to contract
Promotion	The proliferation of a cell with a mutation
Pronation (*Pro-nay-shun*)	Rotation of the hand and forearm – turns the palms down
Proprioceptors (*Pro-pri-oh-cep-tors*)	Sensory receptors that determine the relative position of parts of the body
Propulsion (*Pro-pul-shun*)	The movement of food along the full length of the gastrointestinal tract

Term	Definition
Prosopagnosia (*Pro-sop-ag-no-see-ah*)	Difficulty in recognising faces
Prostaglandins (*Pros-ta-glan-dins*)	A group of lipid compounds with hormone-like effects
Prostate cancer (PCa) (*Pros-tate*)	Malignant tumour of glandular origin in the prostate
Prostate gland	A circular gland, about 4cm (1–2inches) in diameter, that surrounds the urethra and ejaculatory duct adjacent to the bladder and produces prostatic fluid
Prostate specific antigen (PSA)	A serum protein produced by the prostate gland; raised levels may indicate prostate cancer or benign prostatic hyperplasia
Prostate specific membrane antigen (PSMA)	An antigen that facilitates the development of prostate cancer through raising intracellular folate levels. Levels in plasma correlate with severity of cancer and are used as indicators
Prostatic fluid (*Pros-ta-tick*)	The first part of the ejaculate containing most of the sperm
Prostatitis (*Pros-ta-tie-tis*)	Inflammation of the prostate gland
Protease (*Pro-tea-aze*)	An enzyme that breaks down proteins
Proteasome (*Pro-tea-ah-zome*)	Protein complexes which break down proteins by proteolysis
Protein (*Pro-teen*)	Nitrogenous organic compound macronutrient composed of combined polypeptides

Key

Primarily associated with anatomy and physiology

Primarily associated with pathophysiology

Term	Definition
Proteinuria (*Pro-teen-your-e-ah*)	The presence of protein in urine
Proteolysis (*Pro-tea-oh-lie-sis*)	Breakdown of proteins
Proteolytic enzymes (*Pro-tea-oh-lit-ick*)	Enzymes that break down proteins into peptides and amino acids
Proto-oncogene (*Pro-toe-on-ko-jean*)	A gene that codes for proteins that stimulate cell growth (growth factors) and differentiation
Proton pump inhibitors	Drugs that inhibit the activity of pumps transporting hydrogen ions across cell membranes; their main use is to reduce the amount of stomach acid produced
Prothrombin (*Pro-throm-bin*)	A protein that is converted into thrombin for blood clotting – the precursor to thrombin
Protozoa (*Pro-toe-zo-ah*)	A diverse group of mostly motile unicellular eukaryotic organisms (including amoebas, flagellates, ciliates, and sporozoans (e. g. *Plasmodium falciparum*, which causes malaria)) that mostly live parasitically
Pruritus (*Pru-rye-tus*)	Diffuse itching of the skin
Pseudoangiomatous stromal hyperplasia (*Sue-dough-ang-e-oh-mat-us stro-mal high-per-play-see-ah*)	This is a rare and benign breast lesion, one of a group of such lesions, which includes nodular fasciitis. It is a benign proliferation of myofibrils in the stroma
Pseudopods (*Sue-dough-pods*)	Temporary projections of the cell cytoplasm
Pseudopolyps (*Sue-dough-pol-ips*)	Tongue-like projections that resemble polyps

Term	Definition
Psoriasis vulgaris (*So-rye-ah-sis vul-gar-is*)	A T lymphocyte mediated autoimmune skin disorder characterised by focal formation of inflamed, raised skin plaques that constantly desquamate scales as a result of excessive epithelial cell growth
Psoriatic arthritis (PsA) (*Sor-e-ah-tick ar-thry-tis*)	A chronic inflammatory joint disease that is primarily preceded by psoriasis
Puberty (*Pew-ber-tee*)	The process that occurs when changing hormone levels cause development in the reproductive systems to achieve functional reproductive capacity and development of secondary sexual characteristics
Puerperal (*Puer-per-al*)	Related to the period after childbirth
Puerperal fever	Any form of bacterial infection of the female reproductive tract following childbirth or miscarriage
Puerperium (*Puer-per-e-um*)	*See* Postpartum
Pulmonary circulation (*Pul-mon-ar-e*)	Carries the blood between the heart and the lungs permitting exchange of blood gases
Pulmonary embolism (PE)	When a blood borne substance lodges in a branch of the pulmonary artery occluding pulmonary vasculature

Key

Primarily associated with anatomy and physiology

Primarily associated with pathophysiology

Term	Definition
Pulmonary hypertension	High blood pressure in the arterial supply to the lungs; an increase in mean pulmonary arterial pressure (PAPm) greater than 25 mmHg at rest as assessed by right-sided heart catheterisation
Pulmonary oedema	Fluid accumulation in the tissues and alveoli of the lungs
Pulmonary stenosis (*Pul-mon-ar-e sten-oh-sis*)	When there is a narrowing at one or more points between the right ventricle and the pulmonary artery
Pulmonary ventilation (breathing)	The inhalation (inspiration) and exhalation (expiration) of air involving the exchange of air between the atmosphere and the alveoli
Pulp	Core layer of the tooth containing a rich supply of blood and nerves entering from the root
Pulse pressure	The difference between the systolic and diastolic blood pressure that represents the contractile force of the heart
Pupil	The dark circular gap in the iris
Purkinje fibres (*Purr-kin-gee*)	Subdivisions of the AV bundle that pass over the surface of both ventricles, triggering their contraction
Purpura (*Purr-pew-ra*)	Purple spots on the skin secondary to haemorrhage from small blood vessels
Purulent (*Purr-you-lent*)	Producing or containing pus
Pyelonephritis (*Pile-oh-neh-fry-tis*)	Infection/inflammation of the upper urinary tract, affecting the renal parenchyma, i.e. the renal pelvis and medulla (tubules and interstitial tissue)

Term	Definition
Pyloric sphincter (*Pie-lor-ick sphinc-ter*)	Ring of smooth muscle around the opening of the stomach into the duodenum
Pyogenes (*Pie-oh-jeans*)	Gram positive bacteria of the genus *Streptococcus*
Quadriplegia (*Quad-re-plea-gee-ah*)	*See* Tetraplegia
Radiation	The transfer of heat by radiation
Radicular pain (*Ra-dick-u-lar*)	Pain that radiates into a lower extremity directly along the course of a spinal nerve root
Radiotherapy (radiation therapy)	The use of ionising radiation to damage the DNA of cancer cells to delay cell cycle progression and to cause apoptosis
Reactive oxygen species (ROS)	Oxygen-containing molecules formed as a by-product of normal oxygen metabolism and which play important roles in cell signalling and homeostasis
Radius (*Ray-dee-us*)	Shorter of the forearm bones
Receptor (*Re-cept-or*)	A structural component of a sensory neuron, or other cell, that has the ability to respond to a sensory stimulus
Recessive inheritance	When a trait is expressed only when an organism has two recessive alleles (one from each parent) for a gene
Rectocele (*Reck-toe-seal*)	A prolapse of the wall between the rectum and the vagina

Key

Primarily associated with anatomy and physiology

Primarily associated with pathophysiology

Term	Definition
Rectum (*Reck-tum*)	Part of the large intestine which stores faeces until elimination through the anus
Redox reactions	When oxidation and reduction reactions occur in parallel
Reduction	The gain of electrons or a decrease in oxidation state by a molecule, atom, or ion
Reelin (*Ree-lin*)	A glycoprotein that signals migrating neurons and their position in the developing brain
Refeeding syndrome (RFS)	A syndrome that consists of metabolic disturbances following reinstitution of nutrition to people who are severely malnourished, starved or metabolically stressed due to severe illness
Reflex arc	Nerve pathway involved in a reflex action
Refraction (*Ree-frack-shun*)	Bending of light by the lens and cornea
Refractory period (*Ree-frack-toe-ree*)	Period that follows after repolarisation and when the neuron fails to respond to a stimulus of threshold intensity
Regeneration	The ability of the body to replace lost or damaged tissue with the same tissue
Remission	A period of time when a disease process is inactive or less severe
Renal calculi (*Ree-nal kal-cue-lie*)	Kidney stones – polycrystalline aggregates composed of materials that the kidney normally excretes
Renal cortex (*Ree-nal kor-tex*)	The outer section of the kidney between the renal capsule and the renal medulla

Term	Definition
Renal failure	Significant loss of renal function
Renal insufficiency	A decline to about 25% of normal renal function
Renal tubular acidosis (RTA)	A condition where there is impaired renal hydrogen ion excretion (type 1), impaired bicarbonate reabsorption (type 2), or abnormal aldosterone production or response (type 4). Type 3 is no longer included in classifications
Renin (*Re-nin*)	Hormone from the afferent arteriole of the nephron that converts angiotensinogen to angiotensin I
Renin-angiotensin aldosterone System (RAAS) (*Re-nin an-gee-oh-ten-sin al-doss-ter-own*)	A hormonal system that regulates blood volume and systemic vascular resistance
Repolarisation	Restoration of the polarised state of a neuronal cell membrane
Respiratory failure	Failure of the respiratory system to adequately oxygenate the body or to eliminate carbon dioxide from the body
Respiratory tract infections (RTIs)	An infectious disease that can affect any part of the respiratory tract
Respiratory zone	Part of the airway in which gaseous exchange takes place
Restrictive cardiomyopathy	Cardiomyopathy in which the ventricular walls become rigid and inflexible, leading to restricted ventricular filling

Key

Primarily associated with anatomy and physiology

Primarily associated with pathophysiology

Term	Definition
Retching	The muscular (retroperistalsis) event that occurs in vomiting but no stomach contents are expelled
Reticular activating system (RAS) (*Re-tick-u-lar*)	Area of the brain composed of a number of nuclei that connect throughout the forebrain, midbrain and hindbrain and control arousal mechanisms used in maintaining consciousness and awake states essential for selective attention and purposeful responses
Reticular formation (*Re-tick-u-lar*)	A core of nerve cell bodies which extend from the spinal cord up through the medulla, pons and mid-brain to the hypothalamus and thalamus and with connections to the cerebral cortex involved in regulating skeletal muscle tone, autonomic control of the cardiovascular and respiratory systems, and somatic and visceral sensations. It plays a central role in states of consciousness like alertness and sleep
Reticular layer (*Re-tick-u-lar*)	Layer of the dermis below the papillary layer made up of dense irregular connective tissue
Retina (*Ret-in-a*)	A thin transparent membrane attached within the eye that absorbs stray light and is rich in sensory receptors and neural tissue
Retinopathy (*Ret-in-op-ah-thee*)	Disease of the retina that results in impaired vision and blindness
Retrograde (flow) (*Ret-ro-grade*)	Reverse/backward
Retrograde ejaculation	When semen is directed to exit the body through the urethra but is misdirected into the bladder

Term	Definition
Retrovirus (*Ret-ro-viy-rus*)	A virus whose RNA is used inside a host cell to form DNA by means of the enzyme reverse transcriptase
Reverse transcriptase (*Trans-script-ase*)	An enzyme that converts two identical strands of RNA into double stranded DNA once inside the host cell
Rheumatoid arthritis (RA) (*Rue-ma-toid ar-thry-tis*)	A chronic, progressive, systemic autoimmune disease with periods of remission and exacerbation characterised by tenderness and swelling which eventually destroys the synovial joint resulting in disability
Rheumatoid factors (*Rue-ma-toid*)	Autoantibodies involved in rheumatoid arthritis
Rhinitis (*Rye-nigh-tis*)	Inflammation of the mucous membranes of the nose
Rhinorrhoea (*Rye-nor-e-ah*)	Excessive nasal mucus secretion
Ribonucleic acid (RNA) (*Rye-bo-new-kley-ick*)	A nucleic acid molecule that provides a code for the formation of proteins in collaboration with ribosomes
Ribosomes (*Rye-bo-zomes*)	Cellular organelles known as the protein factories. When loose in cytoplasm, they form proteins for use within the cell
Right lymphatic duct	Drains lymph from the right arm and right hand side of the thorax, head and neck, emptying it into the right subclavian vein

Key

Primarily associated with anatomy and physiology

Primarily associated with pathophysiology

Term	Definition
Rods	Photoreceptors responsible for night vision, only seeing black, shades of grey and white
Rotation	Movement of a bone around its longitudinal axis
Rough endoplasmic reticulum (*Rough en-dough-plaz-mick re-tick-you-lum*)	A type of endoplasmic reticulum in the cell that is involved in protein (enzymes and hormones) formation due to containing ribosomes
Ruffini corpuscles (*Rough-e-knee kor-puss-ills*)	General sensory receptors that detect heavy touch, pressure, and stretch
Rugae (*Rue-gay*)	Series of ridges produced by folding of the wall of an organ such as the stomach and bladder
Saccule (*Sack-ule*)	One of the two otolith organs located in the vestibule
Sacral sparing (*Say-kral*)	Preserved movement or sensation in the sacrum due to incomplete spinal cord injury
Sacromeres (*Sack-row-meres*)	Compartments that are the functional unit of the myofibril
Saliva (*Sa-lie-va*)	A slightly acidic liquid composed of water, enzymes, hormones, antibodies, and antimicrobial substances
Salpinges (*Sal-pings*)	*See* Fallopian tube
Salpingitis (*Sal-ping-eye-tis*)	An inflammatory condition of the Fallopian tubes
Salpingo-oophorectomy (*Sal-ping-oh ooh-for-eck-toe-me*)	Removal of the Fallopian tube and ovary from one or both sides of the uterus. Can be combined with hysterectomy when uterus is also removed

Term	Definition
Saltatory conduction (*Sal-ta-toe-ree*)	When neuronal electrical activity jumps between nodes of Ranvier
Sarcoidosis (*Sar-koid-oh-sis*)	A systemic granulomatous disease process that may impact on any organ (in particular the lung) and can mimic other disease processes, especially malignancy or infection
Sarcolemma (*Sar-ko-lem-ah*)	The plasma membrane of the muscle fibre
Sarcoplasm (*Sar-ko-plaz-im*)	The cytoplasm of the muscle fibre
Sarcoplasmic reticulum (SR) (*Sar-ko-plaz-mick re-tick-you-lum*)	A fluid filled sac found in muscle cells that is similar to smooth endoplasmic reticulum. It stores calcium ions and controls their concentration in muscle cells
Satellite cells	Neuroglia that regulate the external chemical environment of neurons, particularly calcium ions
Satiety (*Sah-tie-ah-tee*)	The opposite of hunger, feeling of being full/well fed
Scapula (*Scap-you-la*)	The shoulder blade
Schizophrenia (*Scits-oh-fren-ea*)	A syndrome characterised by signs of psychosis that include paranoid delusions and auditory hallucinations. It can occur at any age, but tends to occur in late adolescence
Schwann cell	A type of neuroglial cell that produces myelin in the peripheral nervous system

Key

Primarily associated with anatomy and physiology

Primarily associated with pathophysiology

Term	Definition
Sclera (*Sclair-ah*)	The white, tough outer layer of the eye composed of connective collagen fibres and contains blood vessels and nerves, providing shape and rigidity to the eye
Scleral venous sinus (*Sclair-al*)	Sinus in the sclera that drains the aqueous humour
Scoliosis (*Sko-lee-oh-sis*)	Abnormal lateral curvature of the spine
Sebaceous glands (*Seh-bay-shus*)	Glands in the skin that produce sebum
Sebum (*See-bum*)	An oily substance that softens & lubricates the skin, prevents hair from becoming brittle, reduces water loss from skin and has antimicrobial properties
Secondary (post-infectious) encephalitis	When a pathogen first infects another part of the body and secondarily enters the brain
Secondary hypertension	When another disorder causes blood pressure to rise
Secondary injury (neurological)	Referring to further damage occurring at cellular level as a result of a primary injury. This can occur over hours or days after the primary injury and includes ischaemia, hypoxia, infection and raised intracranial pressure
Secondary intention	Healing that occurs when there is a tissue deficit between the wound edges requiring a process to fill in and contract the wound area in order to restore tissue integrity
Segmental fracture (*Seg-men-tal*)	When at least two fracture lines isolate a segment of bone
Segmentation (*Seg-men-tae-shun*)	The mixing of the contents of the gut to promote digestion

Term	Definition
Seizure (*See-zure*)	A single episode of electrical neuronal dysfunction, abnormal and excessive excitation and synchronisation of a population of cortical neurons in the brain resulting in an acute, temporary change in neurological functioning
Seizure disorders	Any abnormality generating an electrochemical differential across cell membranes and depolarisation; i.e. an abnormality in an action potential, creating uncontrolled neuronal activity
Self-antigens	An antigen that induces antibody formation in another organism but to which the parent organism is tolerant
Self-tolerance	The ability of the immune system to differentiate between self and foreign antigens
Semicircular canals	Three bony canals in the inner ear filled with endolymph
Semi-lunar valves	Valves at the entrances to the major arteries from the heart
Seminal fluid (*Sem-in-al*)	Semen – fluid that contains sperm and other fluids produced in the male reproductive system during ejaculation
Seminal vesicles	Two blind-ended tubular glands that merge with the vas deferens on the same side to form the ejaculatory duct

Key

Primarily associated with anatomy and physiology

Primarily associated with pathophysiology

Term	Definition
Seminomas (*Sem-e-no-mas*)	Germ cell tumours that are slow growing and contain only seminomatous elements
Sensitisation	A state or condition in which the response to a second or later stimulus is greater than the response to the original. In an immune response, this can lead to hypersensitivity
Sensory division/ system	Division of the PNS that carries sensory information through afferent neurons to the CNS for processing
Sensory receptors	Organs/receptors which convert energy from one form into electrical energy which is transmitted through sensory nerve fibres
Sepsis (*Sep-sis*)	A life-threatening organ dysfunction caused by a dysregulated host response to infection
Septic shock	A subset of sepsis in which profound circulatory, cellular, and metabolic abnormalities are associated with a greater risk of mortality than with sepsis alone
Septum pellucidum (*Sep-tum pel-ew-see-dum*)	Part of the limbic system related to regulating rage, pleasure and mood
Septum primum (*Sep-tum pree-mum*)	When there is tissue growth down in the single atrium of the developing heart in the human embryo. This growth will result in the single atrium being divided into two atria
Septum secundum (*Sep-tum se-cun-dum*)	A tissue growth that descends from the upper wall of the right atrium. After birth, it closes the foramen ovale by fusing with the septum primum

Term	Definition
Serosa (*Ser-oh-sa*)	The outermost layer of lining of a tubular structure which is fibrous and elastic
Serotonin selective reuptake inhibitors (SSRIs) (*Ser-oh-tone-in*)	A type of antidepressant that is believed to increase availability of the neurotransmitter serotonin in the synaptic cleft by limiting its reabsorption (reuptake) into the presynaptic cell. More serotonin is said to be available to bind to the postsynaptic receptor
Serotonin (*Ser-oh-tone-in*)	A neurotransmitter that has a role in memory function, mood and behaviour regulation (anxiety, depression, experience of pain, behaviour, cognition and perception), causes vasoconstriction, and influences gut motility
Serotype (*Sear-oh-type*)	The category of microorganism as characterised by serologic typing
Serous membrane (*Sear-us*)	Double layered membrane that produces serous fluid (pale, watery fluid) between the two layers to provide lubrication
Sertoli cells (*Ser-toll-eye*)	Cells that produce anti-Müllerian hormone and act as the 'nurse' cells for the germ cells in spermatogenesis
Serum amyloid (*See-rum ah-me-loyd*)	A protein capable of starting an immune response and triggering cytokine release
Serum sickness	A systemic allergic reaction to an injection of serum

Key

Primarily associated with anatomy and physiology

Primarily associated with pathophysiology

Term	Definition
Service improvement	The component of public health concerned with the provision of a range of services which contribute to health in different ways (e.g. practice development, service planning, clinical governance)
Sex-linked inheritance	The inheritance of a trait (phenotype) that is determined by a gene located on one of the sex chromosomes (usually the X chromosome)
Sexual orientation	The romantic and/or sexual attraction to another
Sexuality	The interrelationship between the biological, sociocultural and psychological factors that influence the ways in which we experience and express ourselves as sexual beings
Sexually transmitted infections (STIs)	A range of pathogens that can be acquired through sexual contact
Sheehan syndrome (*She-han*)	Hypopituitarism caused by ischaemic necrosis secondary to blood loss and hypovolaemic shock during and after childbirth
Shell temperature	The temperature at or near the surface of the body
Short chain fatty acids (SCFA)	A fatty acid with less than eight carbons
Sight	*See* Vision
Sinoatrial (SA) node (*Sigh-no-a-tree-al*)	Specialised group of autorhythmic cells in the wall of the right atrium which initiate an impulse that spreads across the atria causing them to contract simultaneously
Sinus (*Sigh-nus*)	A cavity within a bone or other tissue

Term	Definition
Sinus arrhythmias (*Sigh-nus a-rith-me-as*)	Arrhythmias that occur as a result of disordered sympathetic stimulation and other homeostatic alterations in temperature, oxygen availability and metabolic changes
Sinus bradycardia (*Sigh-nus brad-e-kar-dee-ah*)	A heart rhythm where the PQRST complex is normal but the ventricular rate is slow (<60 beats per minute)
Sinus tachycardia (*Sigh-nus tack-e-kar-dee-ah*)	A heart rhythm where the PQRST complex is normal but the ventricular rate is fast (>100 beats per minute)
Sinusitis (*Sigh-new-sigh-tus*)	Inflammation/infection of the paranasal sinuses
Sinusoids (*Sigh-new-soids*)	Blood vessels whose walls are incomplete, being lined with highly permeable endothelium
Skeletal muscle fibre	A long cylindrical cell that contains multiple nuclei at the periphery of the fibre
Smegma (*Smeg-ma*)	A waxy substance produced by sebaceous glands in the glans
Smooth endoplasmic reticulum (*En-dough-plaz-mick re-tick-you-lum*)	A type of endoplasmic reticulum in the cell that is involved in steroid (lipid) and carbohydrate metabolism and detoxification
Sodium-potassium pump	A process of active transport that moves potassium ions into, and sodium ions out of, a cell
Somatic (cell) (*So-ma-tick*)	Refers to the cells of the body, excluding germ cells. Any non-reproductive cell

Key

Primarily associated with anatomy and physiology

Primarily associated with pathophysiology

Term	Definition
Somatic nervous system (Motor)	Division of the motor system responsible for voluntary (conscious) control of body movements through stimulating contraction of skeletal muscles
Somatosensation (*So-ma-toe-sen-say-shun*)	Sensations originating mainly in the skin including proprioception, touch and temperature
Sound	Audible vibration of molecules
Spasms	Involuntary movements that often involve multiple muscle groups and joints
Spastic dystonia (*Spa-stick dis-toe-knee-ah*)	Tonic muscle overactivity in the absence of any stimulus
Spasticity (*Spa-tis-ih-tee*)	Increased, involuntary, velocity-dependent muscle tone that causes resistance to movement
Spermatic ducts (*Sper-ma-tick*)	Tubes that take sperm from each testis to the urethra
Spermatocyte (*Sper-ma-toe-site*)	Immature male germ cell, developed from a spermatogonium
Spermatogenesis (*Sper-ma-toe-gen-ih-sis*)	The process of male gamete formation involving creation of a spermatocyte from a spermatogonium, meiotic division of the spermatocyte to create four spermatids that are transformed into spermatozoa
Spermatogonia (*Sper-ma-toe-go-knee-ah*)	Germ cells for sperm formation
Spermatozoa (*Sper-ma-toe-zo-ah*)	Plural of spermatozoon – sperm, the male gamete
Spermatozoon (*Sper-ma-toe-zoon*) Plural spermatozoa	Sperm, the male gamete

Term	Definition
Sphincter (*Sphinc-ter*)	A circular ring of muscle surrounding an opening or tube that can open or close it
Spina bifida (*Spy-na bif-ih-da*)	An open neural tube defect (incomplete closing of backbone and membranes around the spinal cord) and neuro-developmental disorder that originates during embryogenesis, in the first 30 days after fertilisation
Spinal cord	The neural tissue encased within the spine which runs from the medulla to the level of the first or second lumbar vertebrae
Spinal nerves	31 pairs of nerves that carry motor, sensory, and autonomic signals between the spinal cord and the body
Spinal shock	A transient physiological (rather than anatomical) reflex depression of cord function below the level of injury with associated loss of all sensorimotor functions
Spine	The spinal/vertebral column and the mechanical structures of which it is composed - vertebrae and the ligaments and tendons that connect them
Spinocerebellar tracts (*Spy-no-ser-eh-bell-ar*)	Sensory pathways for sensations for muscles and tendons (stretch) to the cerebellum to coordinate skeletal muscle movement
Spiral (torsion) fracture	Fracture that has occurred as a result of a rotating force applied along the axis

Key

Primarily associated with anatomy and physiology

Primarily associated with pathophysiology

Term	Definition
Spongiofibrosis (*Spon-gee-oh-fy-bro-sis*)	When spongiosal tissue is replaced by dense scar tissue that lacks elasticity and contains fibroblasts, forming a urethral stricture
Spongiosal tissue (*Spon-gee-oh-sal*)	Tissue of the corpus spongiosum
Spongy bone	Softer, honeycomb like bone tissue on the inside of bones with spaces containing red and yellow bone marrow and blood vessels
Spontaneous abortion (miscarriage)	The spontaneous loss of a pregnancy before 20 weeks of gestation with the fetus not normally judged as viable
Spontaneous bacterial peritonitis (SBP) (*Per-ih-toe-nigh-tis*)	Bacterial infection in the peritoneum resulting in peritonitis
Spontaneous pneumothorax (*Neu-mo-thor-axe*)	When an air-filled bleb or blister on the surface of the lung ruptures and air enters the pleural cavity
Sprain	Ligament damage
Squamous cell hyperplasia (*Squa-mus cell high-per-play-see-ah*)	A thickened plaque with an irregular surface in the vulva resulting from pruritus leading to rubbing or scratching
Staging (of tumours)	The process of classifying a cancer by its location, growth and spread
SRY	Sex-determining Region of the Y (chromosome) - gene that codes for the production of testis-determining factor (TDF)
Stapedius muscle (*Sta-pee-dee-us*)	Tiny muscle of the ear that dampens large vibrations of the stapes that can occur from loud noises. This protects the oval window and decreases sensitivity of hearing

Term	Definition
Starvation	A decrease in energy intake below the level needed to maintain homeostasis
Static equilibrium (*Eck-we-lib-ree-um*)	Maintenance of body position relative to the force of gravity
Statins (*Sta-tins*)	Drugs that lower LDL (low-density lipoprotein) levels by blocking liver enzymes responsible for making cholesterol
Status asthmaticus (*Sta-tus ass-mat-ick-us*)	A condition where bronchospasm that occurs in asthma has not responded to bronchodilators and or anti-inflammatory drugs
Steatohepatitis (*Stay-ah-toe-hep-ah-tie-tis*)	Inflammatory condition of the liver where there is an accumulation of fat
Steatorrhoea (*Stay-ah-toe-ree-ah*)	Fatty, yellow-grey coloured foul-smelling stools
Steatosis (*Stay-ah-tos-sis*)	Abnormal retention of lipids within hepatocytes
Stem cells	Newly formed cells that have the potential to differentiate into any type of body cell
Stenosis (*Sten-oh-sis*)	Abnormal narrowing of a structure
Stent	A tubular structure placed into a blood vessel to maintain its patency
Sterile	Free from bacteria or other living microorganisms
Sternum (*Ster-num*)	Breast bone

Key

Primarily associated with anatomy and physiology

Primarily associated with pathophysiology

Term	Definition
Steroid hormone	Formed from cholesterol, manufactured in the liver and acquired from the diet
Stevens–Johnson syndrome (SJS)	A rare range of mucocutaneous diseases usually attributable to severe adverse drug reactions. There is widespread inflammation of the epidermis that results in necrosis and sloughing of tissue
Stomach	Bean-shaped sac designed to house food for digestion
Strain (musculoskeletal)	Tendon damage
Strain (microbiological)	A genetic variant or subtype of a microorganism (e.g. virus or bacterium)
Stratum basale (*Stra-tum ba-sal-aa*)	Base layer of the epidermis that has cells which mature and differentiate as they move towards the surface
Stratum corneum (*Stra-tum kor-knee-um*)	Outermost layer of the epidermis where cells are heavily keratinised and waterproof
Stratum granulosum (*Stra-tum gran-you-low-sum*)	Epidermal layer of the skin above the stratum spinosum where keratinisation continues and glycolipids are produced making the cells waterproof
Stratum lucidum (*Stra-tum loo-sid-um*)	Epidermal layer of the skin above the stratum granulosum where cells have clear protoplasm (no organelles) and flattened or no nuclei
Stratum spinosum (*Stra-tum spin-oh-sum*)	Epidermal layer of the skin above the stratum basale that provides structural support to the skin and produces more keratin

Term	Definition
Stress	The biological and psychological response to any adverse stimulus (physical or emotional) that disrupts homeostasis
Stress incontinence	The involuntary passage of urine on effort, physical exertion, coughing or sneezing
Stricture (*Strick-ture*)	The abnormal narrowing of the lumen of a duct, canal or other passage. May be temporary or permanent
Stroke	Gradual or rapid, non-convulsive onset of neurological deficits that fit a known vascular territory and that last for 24 hours or more. There are two types: ischaemic (thromboembolic) and haemorrhagic
Stroke volume	The volume of blood pumped out of each ventricle per heartbeat
Stroma (*Stro-ma*)	The supportive connective tissue of an epithelial organ/tissue/growth
Stromal lesions (*Stro-mal*)	Lesions of connective tissues
Subacute	Refers to conditions which fall between acute and chronic in nature
Subarachnoid haemorrhage (*Sub-ah-rack-noid heem-or-age*)	When there is an arterial rupture and blood flows into the subarachnoid space (and sometimes into the ventricles of the brain). A subarachnoid haemorrhage is usually from the rupture of a cerebral aneurysm

Key

Primarily associated with anatomy and physiology

Primarily associated with pathophysiology

Term	Definition
Subarachnoid space (Sub-ah-rack-noid)	The space between the arachnoid and pia mater through which CSF circulates and within which delicate trabeculae (partitions) of connective tissue extend
Subdural haematoma (Sub-due-ral heem-a-toe-ma)	A collection of blood below the dura above arachnoid membranes of the brain
Sudden arrhythmic death syndrome (SADS) (Aa-rith-mick)	The sudden, untimely death of a young, apparently fit and healthy person due to a cardiac arrhythmia
Sudden cardiac death	When death from SADS is thought to be as a direct result of cardiac disease
Sulci (Sul-ki)	Fissures that divide the brain into lobes
Superoxide dismutase (SOD1) (Sue-per-ox-ide dis-mew-tayze)	An enzyme antioxidant, produced by astrocytes, needed to prevent oxidative stress in a neighbouring motor neuron
Supersaturation of urine	The increased presence in urine of stone components e.g. calcium salts, uric acid, magnesium ammonium phosphate and cystine
Supination (Sue-pin-a-shun)	Rotation of the hand and forearm – turns the palms up
Supplementary prescribers (UK)	Health care professionals permitted to prescribe within the limits of a clinical management plan agreed for a specific group of people by the supplementary prescriber, doctor (independent prescriber) and recipient
Supporting cells (taste)	Cells that lie between taste cells but do not contain taste receptors

Term	Definition
Suppurate (*Sup-per-ate*)	Formation of pus
Supraventricular (*Sue-pra-ven-trick-you-lar*)	Relating to the origin of cardiac impulse being above the ventricles
Surfactant (*Sur-fack-tant*)	A fluid mixture of phospholipids and lipoproteins that lower the surface tension of alveolar fluid to maintain the patency of alveoli
Surgery	When an operative approach, using special techniques manually or with instruments, is used to treat disease, injury or deformity and/or to investigate an illness or improve bodily function or appearance
Suture (*Sue-ture*)	Type of fibrous joint found between the bones of the skull
Sweat	Waste product secreted by sweat glands that contains water, sodium, carbon dioxide, ammonia, urea and other aromatic substances
Symbiotic (*Sim-bi-ot-ick*)	A relationship between different species where both organisms benefit from the presence of the other
Sympathetic nervous system (*Sim-pa-thet-ick*)	A division of the autonomic nervous system that prepares the body for activity (the fight, flight, fright response) through modifying activity of the different systems of the body to increase the supply of nutrients and oxygen for the different activities

Key

Primarily associated with anatomy and physiology

Primarily associated with pathophysiology

Term	Definition
Symphyses (*Sim-phi-ses*)	Type of cartilaginous joints that form permanent joints designed for strength and resilience
Symptomatic (secondary) epilepsy	Epilepsy for which there is a known cause
Synapse (*Sigh-naps (or sin-apps)*)	A specialised intercellular site between two communicating neurons where rapid, highly localised transmission of chemical and electrical signals occurs across a minute gap
Synaptic cleft (*Sigh-nap-tick (or sin-app-tick)*)	Narrow extracellular gap that separates the pre-and post-synaptic membranes of communicating neurons
Synaptogenesis (*Sigh-nap-toe-gen-ih-sis (or sin-app-toe-gen-ih-sis)*)	The creation of synapses between neurons in the nervous system
Synarthroses (*Sin-ar-thro-sis*)	Fixed or unmovable joint
Syncytium (*Sin-sit-e-um*)	Fusion of several cells to form one cell with several nuclei
Synchondroses (*Sin-con-dro-ses*)	Type of cartilaginous joint associated with the growth of bones
Syncope (*Sin-co-pay*)	Partial or complete loss of consciousness with interruption of awareness of oneself and one's surroundings
Syndesmosis (*Sinds-mo-sis*)	Type of fibrous joint found in the lower legs between the distal tibia and fibula and in the forearm between the radius and ulna
Syndrome (*Sin-drome*)	A set of signs and symptoms which occur together and sometimes indicate a specific condition

Term	Definition
Syndrome of inappropriate ADH secretion (SIADH)	A condition in which people develop high levels of, or continuously secrete, ADH; the negative feedback loop that normally controls the amount of ADH secretion fails. As a result, there is increased renal reabsorption of water, resulting in a hypervolaemic, haemodilutional state
Synovial cells (*Sin-oh-ve-al*)	Cells that produce synovial fluid into the capsules of synovial joints
Synovial fluid	A viscous, clear or pale-yellow fluid containing hyaluronic acid and interstitial fluid that forms a thin film over articular capsule surfaces
Synovial joint	Joint with a distinct characteristic of having a space, i.e the synovial cavity, between the ends of the articulating bones
Synovial membrane	Membrane that produces synovial fluid
Synovium (*Sin-oh-ve-um*)	*See* Synovial membrane
Syphilis (*Sif-ih-lus*)	A sexually transmitted infection caused by the bacterium *Treponema pallidum*, an aerobic spirochete bacterium
Syringobulbia (*Ser-in-go-bul-bee-ah*)	A syrinx in the brainstem
Syringomyelia (*Ser-in-go-my-e-lee-ah*)	A syrinx in the upper spinal cord

Key

Primarily associated with anatomy and physiology

Primarily associated with pathophysiology

Term	Definition
Syrinx (*Sir-inks*)	A CSF filled sac in either the brainstem or upper spinal cord
Systemic circulation	The blood supply to the all of the body except the lungs
Systemic inflammatory response syndrome (SIRS)	Systemic activation of the innate immune response regardless of the cause
Systemic lupus erythematosus (SLE) (Lupus) (*Sis-tem-ick loo-pus er-rith-ema-toe-sus*)	An antibody mediated autoimmune disease characterised by chronic inflammation of the tissues of the skin, kidney, blood vessels and other tissues
Systole (*Sis-toe-lay*)	Contraction of the heart muscle during a heartbeat
T helper cells	Type of T cell (lymphocyte) involved in the adaptive immune system that supports activity of other immune cells by releasing cytokines, helping to regulate the immune response.
Tachycardia (*Tack-e-kar-dee-ah*)	Raised heart rate (usually greater than 100 beats per minute)
Tachypnoea (*Tack-e-knee-ah*)	Increased respiratory rate
Tactile corpuscles (*Tack-tile kor-pus-ills*)	General sensory receptors that detect light touch and texture
Tactile discs	General sensory receptors that detect the tactile sensations of light touch, texture, shapes and edges
Tarsal bones (*Tar-sal*)	Bones of the ankle
Tarsal glands	Glands in the eyelid that produce a protective oily lubricant that helps prevent water/tear evaporation from the eye

Term	Definition
Taste (gustatory) cells (*Gus-tae-tory*)	Cells that contain taste hairs that lead into a taste pore with receptors that synapse with a neuron, but are not neurons themselves
Tay–Sachs disease (*Tay-sacks*)	An inherited metabolic disorder caused by deficiency of the enzyme hexosaminidase A that causes a failure to process GM2 ganglioside (a lipid) that accumulates in the brain and other tissues causing damage
T cells	Lymphocytes that secrete immunologically active compounds and assist B cells, are cytotoxic so can destroy foreign cells directly and can self-regulate other T cells by preventing over activity. They also release interleukins which stimulate other lymphocytes and macrophages (from monocytes)
T-cytotoxic cells (*Tee-sigh-toe-tox-ick*)	A T lymphocyte that is antigen-specific and able to source and kill specific types of virus-infected cells
TDF	Testis-determining factor – hormone that initiates the differentiation into male sex organs
Telogen phase (*Tel-oh-gen*)	Final phase of hair growth
Telomerase (*Tel-oh-mer-aze*)	Enzyme that can lengthen the telomere and result in continued division, preventing them from progressively shorting during successive rounds of chromosome replication

Key

Primarily associated with anatomy and physiology

Primarily associated with pathophysiology

Term	Definition
Telomere (*Tel-oh-mear*)	A short length of specific DNA which acts as a buffer against damage and shortening of the chromosome end
Tendons (*Ten-dons*)	Dense fibrous connective tissue that attaches muscle to bone
Teniae coli (*Ten-e-eye ko-lie*)	Three separate longitudinal bands of muscle in the colonic wall
Tenosynovitis (*Ten-oh-sin-oh-vi-tis*)	Inflammation and swelling of the fluid filled sheath (synovium) that surrounds a tendon. Can be infectious or non-infectious
Tension pneumothorax (*Ten-shun new-mo-thor-axe*)	When intrapleural air accumulates under pressure and exceeds atmospheric pressure
Tension type headache (TTH)	Commonest type of headache, episodic or chronic. Some overlap in symptoms with migraine, but rarely disabling or associated with any significant autonomic phenomena
Tensor tympani muscle (*Ten-sor tim-pan-eye*)	Tiny muscle connected to the ossicles that limits movement and increases tension on the eardrum to prevent damage to the inner ear from loud noises
Teratogenic (*Ter-ah-toe-gen-ick*)	Relating to any substance that can disrupt the healthy development of an embryo or fetus
Teratoma (*Ter-ah-toe-ma*)	A germ cell tumour composed of different types of tissues
Teratozoospermia (*Ter-ah-toe-zoo-sper-me-ah*)	Sperm with abnormalities
Terminal cisterns (*Sis-terns*)	Open-ended sacs of the sarcoplasmic reticulum that sit against the sides of T tubules

Term	Definition
Tertiary intention	Healing that occurs when a wound is intentionally kept open to allow oedema or infection to resolve or to permit removal of exudate
Testicular torsion (*Tes-tick-you-lar tor-shun*)	When there is twisting of the testis on the spermatic cord, obstructing the blood flow to the testis
Tetraplegia (*Tet-ra-plee-gee-ah*)	Injury to the cervical spinal cord with associated loss of motor and/or sensory function in all four extremities
Thalamus (*Thal-a-mus*)	Relay centre for nervous impulses moving to and from the cerebrum
Thalassaemia (*Thal-a-see-me-ah*)	Group of conditions in which the rate of formation of haemoglobin is reduced but the structure is normal
T helper cells	A T lymphocyte that provides assistance to other cells in the immune response by recognising antigens and secreting cytokines to activate T and B cells
Thermoceptors (*Ther-mo-sep-tors*)	Sensory receptors that respond to temperature
Thermogenesis (*Ther-mo-gen-ih-sis*)	The production of heat
Thermoregulation (*Ther-mo-reg-you-lay-shun*)	The regulation of body temperature
Thermosensation (*Ther-mo-sen-say-shun*)	Perception of temperature

Key

Primarily associated with anatomy and physiology

Primarily associated with pathophysiology

Term	Definition
Thoracic duct (*Tho-ra-sick*)	Lymph vessel that returns lymph collected from legs, pelvic region and abdominal cavity, the left arm and the left-hand side of the thorax, head and neck to the circulatory system by emptying into the left subclavian vein
Thrombin (*Throm-bin*)	An enzyme in the blood that has a role in coagulation by converting fibrinogen to fibrin
Thrombocytes (*Throm-bo-sites*)	Very small discs without nuclei that secrete clotting factors (pro-coagulants), vasoconstricting agents to induce vascular spasm, and clump together in platelet plugs. They also dissolve old blood clots, destroy bacteria by phagocytosis, secrete chemical agents, attract neutrophils and monocytes to infected sites by chemical messengers and promote mitosis in fibroblasts and smooth muscle
Thrombocythaemia (*Throm-bo-sigh-thee-me-ah*)	A disorder in which excess thrombocytes are produced
Thrombocytopenia (*Throm-bo-sigh-toe-pee-knee-ah*)	When there is a reduced number of thrombocytes being formed, resulting in a low level of platelets in the blood
Thrombolysis (*Throm-bo-lie-sis*)	When a thrombus is dissolved using medication
Thrombosis (*Throm-bo-sis*)	Formation/presence of a blood clot in a blood vessel
Thyroid storm (*Thigh-roid*)	*See* Thyrotoxic crisis
Thyrotoxic crisis (*Thigh-row-tox-ick*)	An acute, life-threatening hypermetabolic state secondary to excessive levels of thyroid hormone in people with thyrotoxicosis

Term	Definition
Thyrotoxicosis (*Thigh-row-tox-e-ko-sis*)	The clinical effects experienced due to an excess of thyroid hormones in the bloodstream (hyperthyroidism)
Tibia (*Tib-e-ah*)	The shin bone – the stronger of the two bones in the lower leg
Tidal volume (*Tie-dal*)	The amount of air that moves with one breath
T lymphocyte (*Tea-limph-oh-site*)	Type of lymphocyte that has a central role in cell-mediated immunity
Tonic (*Ton-ick*)	Phase of a seizure in which there is increased tone of voluntary muscle
Tonicity (of a fluid) (*Ton-iss-ih-tee*)	The force exerted by osmotically active particles within a fluid
Tonsillitis (*Ton-sil-eye-tis*)	Inflammation of the tonsils
Tophi (*Toe-fee*)	Hard white nodules formed of deposits of crystalline uric acid and other substances
Topical (*Top-ick-al*)	Relating to the application of medicinal products directly to a part of the body (e.g. to the skin)
Toxic epidermal necrolysis (TEN) (*Tox-ick epp-e-der-mal neh-krol-ih-sis*)	*See* Stevens–Johnson syndrome (SJS)
Trabeculae (*Tra-beck-you-lay*)	Supporting columns of connective tissue within an organ/structure

Key

Primarily associated with anatomy and physiology

Primarily associated with pathophysiology

Term	Definition
Trachea (*Tra-key-ah*)	A tubular passageway of connective tissue and smooth muscle reinforced with C-shaped rings of hyaline cartilage extending from the larynx to the bronchial tubes to bring air to and from the lungs
Transamination (*Trans-am-in-nay-shun*)	The transfer of the nitrogen element from one molecule to another to form an amino acid
Transcellularly (*Trans-cell-you-lar-lee*)	Referring to penetration of a cell and travelling through it
Transcription (*Trans-crip-shun*)	The first step of gene expression where a particular segment of DNA is copied into RNA
Transcytosis (*Tran-sigh-toe-sis*)	Transport of large molecules by capturing them in vesicles, carrying them across a cell, and exporting them out the other side
Transfer protein	A cell membrane protein that facilitates the transport of a substance across that membrane
Transient ischaemic attack (TIA) (*Tran-see-ant ih-skee-mick*)	A temporary focal loss of neurological function (less than 24 hours) caused by ischaemia
Transients (*Tran-see-ants*)	Microorganisms that get incorporated briefly into the microbiota from the diet or environment but do not remain long and are unable to colonise the body
Translocation (*Trans-low-kay-shun*)	The movement of something from one place to another, e.g. bacteria from the gastrointestinal tract into the circulation
Transmural (*Trans-mew-ral*)	Occurring across the entire wall of an organ/structure

Term	Definition
Transposition of the Great Arteries (*Trans-po-zish-shun*)	When the aorta arises from the right ventricle and the pulmonary artery from the left ventricle, i.e. the opposite to the normal location of these vessels
Transverse fracture	Fracture in which the fracture line is perpendicular to the shaft of the bone
Transverse T tubules	Small tubules that run transversely through striated muscle fibres and through which action potentials are transmitted from the sarcoplasm into the fibre
Traumatic subarachnoid haemorrhage (*Traw-mat-ick sub-ah-rack-noid heem-or-age*)	When rotational, stretching and tearing forces cause arteries to rupture with haemorrhage in the subarachnoid space
T regulatory cells	A T lymphocyte that suppresses other lymphocytes' activity and controls immune responses
Trichomoniasis (*Trick-oh-mon-eye-ih-sis*)	An STI caused by the protozoan *Trichomonas vaginalis*, an anaerobic flagellated protozoan
Trigeminal neuralgia (TN) (*Try-gem-in-al new-ral-gee-ah*)	A form of neuralgia that occurs largely from compression of the trigeminal nerve or from another structural abnormality that triggers the nerve
Triglycerides (*Try-gliss-er-ides*)	Type of fat composed of one molecule of glycerol joined with three fatty acid molecules

Key

Primarily associated with anatomy and physiology

Primarily associated with pathophysiology

Term	Definition
Trimester (*Try-mess-ter*)	A three-month period of pregnancy
Trisomy (*Try-so-me*)	When there are three copies of a specific chromosome instead of the normal two
Trophoblasts (*Tro-pho-blasts*)	Cells that form the outer layer of the blastocyst
Trypsin (*Trip-sin*)	A digestive enzyme which breaks down proteins in the small intestine
Trypsinogen (*Trip-sin-oh-gen*)	The inactive precursor of trypsin
Tuberculosis (*Two-bur-kew-low-sis*)	A highly contagious infection caused by *Mycobacterium tuberculosis* (MTB) (an acid-fast bacillus), usually affecting the lungs but may invade other body systems
Tumour (*Chu-mur* or *Tu-mor*)	A swelling which can result from various conditions including inflammation and trauma
Tumour markers	Biochemical substances produced by some cancer cells
Tumour necrosis factor (TNF) (*Chu-mur neh-crow-sis*)	A cytokine, secreted by macrophages, that induces cell death of mutated cells
Tumour Nodes Metastasis (TNM) system (*Meh-ta-sta-sis*)	International cancer classification system
Tumour suppressor genes (TSG)	Genes that control growth inhibitory signals
Tunica albugenia (*Tew-nick-ah al-bew-gee-knee-ah*)	Fibrous envelope covering the penile corpora cavernosa that creates partitions between seminiferous tubules
Tunica externa (*Tew-nick-ah ex-ter-nah*)	Outer fibrous layer of blood vessels

Term	Definition
Tunica interna (*Tew-nick-ah in-ter-nah*)	Inner, smooth layer of blood vessels
Tunica media (*Tew-nick-ah me-dee-ah*)	Middle muscular layer of blood vessels
Tunica vaginalis (*Tew-nick-ah vaj-in-ah-lis*)	The serous membrane that covers the anterior and lateral surfaces of the testes
Tympanic cavity (*Tim-pan-ick*)	Air filled cavity behind the eardrum that connects to the nasopharynx by the Eustachian tube (or auditory tube)
Tympanic membrane	A thin semi-transparent partition between the auditory canal and the middle ear
Tyrosinaemia (*Tie-row-sin-e-me-ah*)	A genetic disorder characterised by impairment in the process of breaking down the amino acid tyrosine, a building block of most proteins. This results in high levels of tyrosine in the blood
Ubiquitin (*You-bic-wit-in*)	A small protein found in all cells of the body which affects proteins in many ways
Ubiquitination (*You-bic-wit-in-a-shun*)	When a protein has ubiquitin attached to it, signalling that the protein is to be transported to a proteasome for degradation, where it affects their activity, and promotes or prevents protein interactions
Ulcer (*Ul-ser*)	An open sore on an external or internal surface of the body (organ or tissue), resulting from necrosis that accompanies inflammatory, infectious or malignant processes

Key

Primarily associated with anatomy and physiology

Primarily associated with pathophysiology

Term	Definition
Ulcerative colitis (UC) (*Ul-ser-ah-tiv ko-lie-tis*)	A non-specific inflammatory condition of the colon and rectum
Ulna (*Ul-nah*)	The longest of the forearm bones
Umbilical cord (*Um-bil-ick-al (or um-bi-lie-kal)*)	The vascular cord that connects an embryo or fetus to the placenta
Unresponsive wakefulness syndrome (UWS)	*See* Vegetative state (VS)
Unstable angina (*An-ji-nah*)	Chest pain secondary to reduced blood flow to the coronary arteries caused by unstable plaques that rupture or erode, exposing the plaque core to blood flow. In unstable angina, the person will experience pain at rest as a result of myocardial ischaemia secondary to insufficient oxygen to meet myocardial tissue demands
Uraemia (*Yur-e-me-ah*)	High blood urea
Uraemic syndrome (*Yur-e-mick sin-drome*)	A syndrome characterised by increased blood serum levels of urea and creatinine alongside neurological changes, nausea, vomiting, anorexia and fatigue
Urea (*Yur-e-ah*)	Formed in the liver from amino acids, this is the primary nitrogenous waste product of protein catabolism (breakdown)
Ureters (*Yur-ih-ters*)	Pair of tubes which collect urine from the calyces of the kidneys and drain it into the bladder by peristalsis
Urethra (*Yur-e-thra*)	Tube that carries urine from the bladder (and semen in men) to the external urinary meatus for elimination from the body

Term	Definition
Urethral stricture (*Yur-e-thral strick-ture*)	A narrowing of the urethral lumen; it may be obstructive or disruptive to flow through the urethra or the person may be asymptomatic
Urethritis (*Yur-ih-thry-tis*)	Inflammation of the urethra
Urethrocele (*Yur-e-thro-seal*)	When part of the vaginal wall fused to the urethra descends and causes disruption of continence
Urethroplasty (*Yur-e-thro-plas-tee*)	Repair of a damaged urethra
Urethrotomy	Incision of the fibrotic scar tissue in the urethra
Urge incontinence	The involuntary loss of urine accompanied by, or immediately preceded by, urgency
Urinary incontinence	The loss of voluntary control of the bladder resulting in involuntary leakage of urine
Urinary meatus (*Mee-a-tus*)	External urethral opening
Urinary oxalates (*Ox-ah-lates*)	Chemicals in the urine which can form kidney stones
Urticaria (*Ur-te-care-e-ah*)	A skin reaction characterised by fluid filled blisters known as wheals and surrounded by an area of redness known as flares
Uterine prolapse (*You-ter-ine pro-laps*)	When the main supportive ligaments for the uterus are stretched and the uterus bulges down into the vagina

Key

Primarily associated with anatomy and physiology

Primarily associated with pathophysiology

Term	Definition
Uterus (*You-ter-us*)	The womb
Utricle (*You-trick-ul*)	One of the two otolith organs located in the vestibule (inner ear)
Uveitis (*You-ve-eye-tis*)	Inflammation of the uvea, the middle layer of the eye between the sclera and the retina
Uvula (*You-vue-la*)	Small, fleshy, conical body projecting downward from the middle of the soft palate
Vaccination (*Vack-sin-a-shun*)	The administration of a vaccine (antigenic material) – a biological preparation that stimulates an individual's immune system to develop adaptive immunity to a specific infectious disease
Vacuolating toxin (*Vack-you-oh-lay-ting*)	A toxin involved in *Helicobacter pylori* pathogenesis
Vagina (*Vah-ji-nah*)	The fibromuscular tube which runs from the cervix to the opening to the external genitalia
Vaginitis (*Vag-in-eye-tis*)	Inflammation of the vagina with discharge, itching, burning, redness and swelling
Valency (*Vay-len-see*)	The combining power of an element determined by the number of hydrogen atoms it can transfer or combine with
Vaptans (*Vap-tans*)	Oral vasopressin antagonists
Variable expression	The extent to which a phenotype is expressed to different degrees among individuals with the same genotype
Varicocele (*Var-ick-oh-seal*)	A vascular abnormality of the testicular venous drainage system whereby these veins become abnormally dilated and tortuous

Term	Definition
Vascular endothelial growth factor (VEGF) (*Vas-cue-lar en-dough-thee-lee-al*)	A signal protein that stimulates the proliferation of vascular endothelial cells, contributing to blood vessel development
Vascular tunic (*Vas-cue-lar tew-nick*)	Section of the eye made up of the choroid, ciliary body and iris
Vasculitis (*Vas-cue-lie-tis*)	Inflammation of a blood vessel(s)
Vasoconstriction (*Vay-zo-kon-strick-shun*)	Narrowing of the lumen of blood vessels through contraction of the smooth muscle within the vessel walls
Vasodilation (*Vay-zo-die-lay-shun*)	Widening of the lumen of blood vessels through relaxation of the smooth muscle within the vessel walls
Vasopressors (*Vay-zo-press-ors*)	Drugs/agents that cause vasoconstriction
Vasospasm (*Vay-zo-spaz-im*)	Arterial spasm that leads to vasoconstriction
Vegetative state (VS) (*Veg-eh-tay-tive*)	A disorder of consciousness where a person appears awake but displays no behavioural signs of awareness; a sleep–wake cycle is present and there may be reflexive and spontaneous behaviours but not in response to stimuli
Veins	Blood vessels that carry blood back towards the heart
Ventilation (*Ven-til-a-shun*)	The amount of air that enters the alveoli

Key

Primarily associated with anatomy and physiology

Primarily associated with pathophysiology

Term	Definition
Ventilation/perfusion (V/Q) mismatch	Abnormal ventilation/perfusion ratio, e.g. when areas of the lungs are better perfused by blood than they are ventilated (e.g. lack of alveoli), or better ventilated than perfused with blood (e.g. lack of blood supply to a well-ventilated lung with sufficient alveoli)
Ventricle (brain) (*Ven-trick-al*)	Chambers of the brain filled with CSF
Ventricle (heart) (*Ven-trick-al*)	Lower, larger chamber of the heart, of which there are two, that receive blood from the atria for pumping out around the body. The right ventricle pumps blood to the lungs and the left out to the rest of the body
Ventricular fibrillation (VF) (*Ven-trick-you-lar fib-ril-ay-shun*)	A disorder with uncoordinated ventricular activation that results in deterioration of ventricular function; the ventricles fibrillate (i.e. quivering movement caused by uncoordinated contraction) and therefore do not contract sufficiently to produce cardiac output
Ventricular septal defects (VSDs) (*Ven-trick-you-lar sep-tal*)	Openings in the ventricular septum enabling blood to shunt from one side to the other
Ventricular tachycardia (VT) (*Ven-trick-you-lar tacke-e-kar-dee-ah*)	When the cardiac impulse is generated from increased automaticity at a single point in either the left or the right ventricle that leads to a fast, organised rhythm
Venules (*Ven-youles*)	Small veins
Vertebrae (*Ver-te-bray*)	Small bones forming the spine

Term	Definition
Vertex presentation (*Ver-tecks*)	When the head of the fetus descends into the pelvis
Very low density lipoproteins (VLDLs) (*Lie-po-pro-teens*)	Precursors to LDLs, these lipoproteins have their triglycerides removed in adipocytes and become LDLs
Vesicle (*Veh-sic-el*)	A cellular organelle comprised of a fluid enclosed by a lipid bilayer membrane, within which substances can be stored for secretion
Vesiculation (*Veh-sic-you-lay-shun*)	Blistering
Vestibular apparatus (*Veh-stib-you-lar ah-par-ah-tus*)	Organ of balance consisting of the vestibule and the semicircular canals
Vestibule (ear) (*Veh-sti-bule*)	One of the two major parts of the vestibular apparatus, consists of a pair of membranous sacs, the saccule and utricle
Vestibule (nasal) (*Veh-sti-bule*)	Anterior portion of nasal cavity
Vestibule (vulvar) (*Veh-sti-bule*)	Part of the vulva between the labia minora into which the urethra and vagina open
Villi (*Vil-eye*)	Minute finger-shaped processes of the mucous membrane of the small intestine
Viron (*Vi-ron*)	The extracellular infective form of a complete virus particle consisting of a single or double strand of RNA or DNA surrounded by a protein coat

Key

Primarily associated with anatomy and physiology

Primarily associated with pathophysiology

Term	Definition
Virus (*Vi-rus*)	Any of a wide variety of mostly pathogenic microorganisms consisting of a single nucleic acid chain surrounded by a protein coat, capable of replication only within another living cell
Viscosity (*Vis-kos-it-e*)	The thickness of a fluid; a measure of its resistance to flow
Viscerosensation (*Vis-ser-oh-sen-say-shun*)	Sensations originating in internal organs including pain, palpitations and spasms
Vision	The conversion of electromagnetic radiation to electrochemical energy in order to produce images of our surroundings
Vitamin D	A lipophilic vitamin and hormone synthesised in the skin by the conversion of 7dehydrocholesterol to vitamin D by ultraviolet radiation from the sun
Vitiligo (*Vih-ti-lie-go*)	A skin depigmentation condition where patches of skin progressively lose pigmentation, characterised by white skin with sharp, distinct margins
Vitreous humour (*Vih-tree-us hue-mor*)	The clear, gel-like substance filling the eyeball behind the lens
Volkmann's canals	Small channels in the bone that transmit blood vessels from the periosteum into the bone
Volume-responsive (prerenal) AKI	Acute kidney injury (AKI) as a result of decreased blood supply to the kidneys (glomeruli and renal tubule undamaged)
Vomiting	*See* Emesis
Vulva (*Vul-va*)	External genitals of the female

Term	Definition
Vulvodynia (*Vul-vo-din-e-ah*)	Vulval pain or burning sensation without visible lesions
Water of oxidation	Water created through metabolic reactions
Waterhouse–Friderichsen syndrome	Adrenal gland failure due to haemorrhage into the adrenal glands, commonly caused by severe bacterial infection
Wernicke's aphasia (*Ver-nicks a-phase-e-ah*)	Fluent aphasia – impairment of the ability to grasp the meaning of spoken words. Person can usually produce correct speech but sentences often do not connect well. Reading and writing usually severely impaired
White matter	Grouping of nerve cell axons
Wolman disease (*Vol-man*)	A severe type of lysosomal acid lipase deficiency that results in impaired metabolism of lipids
Zona fasciculata (*Zone-ah va-sick-you-lah-ta*)	Layer of the adrenal gland that secretes glucocorticoid hormones, including cortisol
Zona glomerulosa (*Zone-ah gloh-mer-you-low-sah*)	Layer of the adrenal gland that secretes aldosterone
Zona reticularis (*Zone-ah reh-tick-you-lar-iss*)	Layer of the adrenal gland that produces androgens
Zygote (*Zi-goat*)	The name given to the fertilised egg cell formed by the fusion of a sperm cell and an ovum

Key

Primarily associated with anatomy and physiology

Primarily associated with pathophysiology

PART 3
NOTES

Use this space to add your own terms and definitions as you encounter them. For complex and unfamiliar words use the dissection method to break the term down into its component parts.

Notes

....

....

....

....

....

....

....

....

....

....

Notes

Notes

Notes

Notes

Notes

Notes

Notes

Notes

Notes

Notes

Notes

Notes

Notes